KU-449-918

WHAT WILL **REALLY** HELP YOU
LEAD A MORE JOYFUL LIFE?

THE

HOW

OF

Happy

ARIANE SHERINE
AND DAVID CONRAD

ROBINSON

ROBINSON

First published in Great Britain in 2022 by Robinson

13 5 7 9 10 8 6 4 2

Copyright © Ariane Sherine and David Conrad, 2022

The moral right of the authors has been asserted.

All rights reserved.
No part of this publication may be reproduced, stored in a retrieval system,
or transmitted, in any form, or by any means, without the prior permission in writing
of the publisher, nor be otherwise circulated in any form of binding or cover other than
that in which it is published and without a similar condition including this condition
being imposed on the subsequent purchaser.

A CIP catalogue record for this book
is available from the British Library.

ISBN: 978-1-47214-390-7

Typeset in Garamond Premier Pro by SX Composing DTP, Rayleigh, Essex
Printed and bound in Great Britain by Clays Ltd, Elcograf S.p.A.

Papers used by Robinson are from well-managed forests
and other responsible sources.

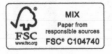

Robinson
An imprint of
Little, Brown Book Group
Carmelite House

FLINTSHIRE
SIR Y FFLINT WITHDRAWN

C29 0000 0917 909

Askews & Holts	07-Nov-2022
158	£14.99
FLIMOLD	

C29 0000 0917 909

A**r**... **e Sherine** is a comedy writer and journalist. Her work has appeared in, ... ong others, the *Guardian*, *The Sunday Times*, the *Observer* and the *I*... *lent*, and she has worked as a scriptwriter for the BBC, Channel ... TV. She is about to launch her debut solo pop album *Bitter* under ... ist name Ariane X. Written, produced and performed by Ariane, ... ctropop and dance tracks will appeal to fans of Depeche Mode, ... Étienne and Garbage. *Bitter* is available to stream on Spotify, Apple ... and all other streaming services from April 2023.

... **l Conrad** (MA; MSc; MPH; FFPH) is a Consultant in Public ... alth. Together with Professor Alan White from Leeds Beckett ... iversity, he has co-edited three books for health professionals – *Men's H*... *: How to Do It* (Radcliffe, 2007); *Promoting Men's Mental Health* (... iffe, 2010) and *Sports-Based Health Interventions: Case Studies* ... *Around the World* (Springer, 2016). He also co-edited the public ... h textbook *Health Protection: Principles and Practice* (Oxford ... iversity Press, 2016) and has published papers in several peer-reviewed ... ientific journals.

Also by Ariane Sherine and David Conrad

How to Live to 100

Talk Yourself Better (by Ariane Sherine)

For Lily, as ever, with all our love

Contents

THE
HOW
OF
Happy

Introduction

Happiness: as elusive as a working inkjet printer, and as slippery as an eel covered in baby oil. If you chase it, it runs away faster than a cat when you're trying to give it a bath.

But we all carry on chasing happiness, as a life without joy is like a Jacuzzi with no water in – sure, it technically exists, but it's zero fun. So we strive for pleasure and contentment, sometimes searching in all the wrong places.

Luckily for you, you're holding a book full of the secrets to happiness. And not some spurious bollocks Law-of-Attraction-based self-help tome, either, where they tell you to just 'think of what you want' in order to get it (I've been thinking about marrying Mark Ruffalo for a long time now, and he still doesn't know I exist).

No: this is as evidence-based a guide to happiness as you can get. My co-author David has painstakingly rooted out fifty recent studies from scientific journals, like a pig rooting out expensive truffles from the ground. (No, David, I'm not calling you a pig. Please don't stop talking to me again, David. David, where are you going?!)

Each 'truffle', aka study, has its own chapter, looking at a different subject which has been linked to happiness. It starts with David's lofty academic summary of a piece of research on the topic, full of sexy authority and gravitas, followed by a 'Happiness Hint' for applying the findings to your own life. (David's single by the way, ladies, so hit him up and he might make you very happy.) After his bit, I come in with the fun part and tell you what I think of it.

The chapters are split into four sections, each with its own theme: 'Family and relationships', 'Work, money and spending', 'Health and beauty' and 'Outlook on life'. All the research studies described have been published in fancy academic peer-reviewed journals, and we've included a reference at the end of each chapter so you can see where they came from.

This scientific guide is much more likely to help you than self-help books on happiness confected from woo and fairy dust, because it's based on hard evidence, not fiction pulled from the woolly brain of some self-described guru. It contains a broad and interesting range of topics, and you can go and read the studies for yourself if you like (though they're not as interesting as this book, I promise).

What I'll tell you here, which the authors of snake-oil tomes never will, is that this isn't an exhaustive list of all the things that might determine happiness. Scientists are conducting new studies all the time, and there are plenty of other things being looked at in the field of happiness research which we haven't been able to capture in this book.

In addition, it's worth bearing in mind that a single study rarely gives us a definitive answer to a research question. All studies have their strengths and limitations, depending on the methods used. Researchers, for example, often struggle to recruit a representative sample of the general population to take part in their studies, making it hard to tell how universally applicable their findings are.

Another challenge is being able to determine whether two things are merely correlated, or whether one can truly be said to cause the other. It's much more common to find studies which only demonstrate correlations, simply because of the complexity and resources needed to undertake studies which can prove causality.

And as a result of the constraints faced by researchers and the different methods applied, two studies aiming to answer the same question can produce conflicting findings. We've tried to acknowledge some of the key limitations of the studies included in the book as we've gone along, and to be open about how confidently we can apply their findings in everyday life.

However, before you put this book down in disgust and pick up another, it's a bloody good start on the road to happiness, busting a lot of myths you might have come across when trying to find joy in your own life. We reckon you'll find each of the chapters insightful, but we don't expect that every reader will be able to apply all of the findings from these studies in their own lives – or at least, not all at once. Some of the messages and tips might seem a little incompatible, but they aren't intended as a rigid checklist of essential requirements to achieve happiness. You can pick the ones that seem most applicable and practical for you right now and keep the rest in your happiness toolkit for another day – or pass them on to someone else!

Each study has the year it was published* and the country**. You won't care about the asterisks, but David wanted me to tell you about them, and I should as he's already upset about the pig thing.

Lastly, there are celebrity contributions in this book from such luminaries as Derren Brown, Stewart Lee, Jeremy Vine, Rosie Holt, Femi Oluwole, Sanjeev Kohli, Arthur Smith, Count Binface, Bec Hill, Jon Holmes, Mhairi McFarlane and many more, explaining what makes them happy personally and giving you their best advice on happiness.

Now go and read the book and apply its principles to your life, so you can cheer up before it's too late. Go on. Shoo! Or I'll break your inkjet printer.

---

* Occasionally this differs from the reference at the end of the chapter, as academic journals sometimes publish studies online before they come out in print, just in case you're thinking, 'Uh?!'

** The place/s from which the study data was collected isn't always the same as the country where the study was written, as researchers often collect or use data gathered by others from different countries. No idea why you'd care, but I've promised to tell you this, and also that 'various' means data from more than three countries was included, and 'unspecified' means this info wasn't made explicit in the study report. There you go, isn't your life so much better for knowing this?

Part 1: Family and relationships

Being around happy people

Research study 📁

Title: Is Happiness Infectious?

Year: 2017

Country: China

Using data from a national survey of people in rural China, this study attempted to establish whether happiness is infectious. The data was collected in 2002 by China's National Bureau of Statistics from randomly selected households across twenty-two provinces.

The survey questionnaire covered a range of topics, including a section on subjective wellbeing. One member of each household was asked 'How happy are you nowadays?' with a range of five options from 'very happy' to 'not at all happy'. The respondents were also asked about which people they tended to compare themselves with. Almost 70% said that they compared themselves with their neighbours and others in the village, giving the researchers confidence that the right place to look for any evidence of happiness spreading from person to person was within individual villages.

Complex analysis was required to search for signs in the data that an individual respondent's happiness was dependent on the happiness of their village acquaintances. Demonstrating a correlation between the two wasn't enough on its own, as this might simply have been due to having certain experiences or characteristics in common which affect happiness, such as village amenities or employment.

The researchers concluded that there was some evidence of a causal link between a person's level of individual happiness and that of the people they compared themselves with. They also described how this effect is in apparent conflict with the established link between relative income and happiness. Those with higher incomes tend to be happier, but we tend to be less happy when the income of our peers is relatively higher than our own. If happiness is truly infectious, when one of our peers becomes happier due to achieving a greater income we should also become happier as their happiness spreads to us. But at the same time, we would lose some happiness because we would now also be relatively worse off financially. The researchers suggested that the overall balance of these effects may depend on the extent to which our 'happiness comparator' group and 'income comparator' group overlap.

The findings of this study are interesting, but we need to be cautious about using them to make generalisations. Most people living in rural areas of China have very low incomes and live in villages with an average size of 450 households. The houses are typically grouped together, with the village being the centre of social life for its inhabitants. Studies would need to be conducted in different locations to know whether the same results would be seen in other types of setting, such as a European city neighbourhood.

Happiness hint ☑

Hang around with happy people (preferably ones whose happiness isn't entirely due to earning more money than you).

I don't buy this idea that happiness is necessarily catching – it can often lead to jealousy and envy. I had two close female friends who went full-on Othello on me just because I got married and got a book deal. They wanted to be in the same situation, and found my personal and professional success impossible to handle.

Which is all a bit nuts, because I'm not exactly rivalling Michelle Obama in the success stakes.

I felt very sad for these friends, and also extremely frustrated and miserable, because the situation was out of my control (I mean, unless I told my husband and publisher to piss off, and what kind of maniac does that to appease their friends?!).

Friends are meant to be happy for each other – that's the theory, anyway, though I reckon Morrissey was spot-on with his song 'We Hate It When Our Friends Become Successful' (yes, I'm aware he's a mad buffoon now, but that doesn't mean he can't ever be right).

Eventually, we parted ways acrimoniously and don't even exchange Christmas cards these days (me and my ex-friends, not me and Mozza). I reckon the only way I'm getting a card from them is if it's filled with their own shit.

I occasionally miss our former closeness and girly chats, but am also relieved to be free of their toxicity and rancour. I never gave them anything but kindness, and no one should be made to feel bad for achieving things that don't hurt other people.

The study would also suggest that being around depressing people is depressing! Whooda thunk?

I found this out early on. I was clinically depressed in my late teens and early twenties, and twice tried to take my own life (this is a cheery start to the book, isn't it?).

Because of this, a friend dumped me as I brought her down (which made me even sadder, as she was literally the coolest person I'd ever met. She lived in a squat and smoked weed, how much cooler can you get?!).

Later on, I would avoid miserable people myself because I felt so low after speaking to them.

While it doesn't seem fair that the unhappiness of unhappy people is exacerbated because everyone shuns them, it also stands to reason that no one wants to feel low. Life is tough enough with random circumstance biting you in the arse every so often, without having to deal with other people's misery on top of it all.

To echo the study above, I've also noticed that angry people get even angrier when you earn more than them. It compounds their sense of life's unfairness: not only are they unhappy but they're not getting their fair share economically either. Which then makes you feel guilty and decide to avoid them, so nobody wins.

Conversely, I love hanging out with my cheery adopted grandad, John, whom I call John Bon Jovial because he's just so happy. Yes, he's a Tory Brexiteer and makes all the worst dad jokes (Me: 'I'll join you'; Him: 'I didn't know I was coming apart!'), but his happiness and enthusiasm are as catchy as Covid (which he actually gave me last Christmas. Thanks, Grandad!).

And this upbeat outlook may be why he's reached his seventies in perfect health despite barely eating any fruit or veg. He even had asymptomatic Covid, while I was coughing up my lungs like a frog with emphysema.

I don't know if the fact that he's also totally skint adds to my happiness, but I'd like to think not.

Reference:
Knight J., Gunatilaka R., Is Happiness Infectious? *Scott J Polit Econ*. 2017;64(1):1–24. doi:10.1111/sjpe.12105

Having friends you matter to

Research study 🗁

Title: I Matter to My Friend, Therefore I am Happy: Friendship, Mattering, and Happiness

Year: 2010

Country: USA

Lots of research has demonstrated that having good quality, close friendships is associated with happiness, but exactly why this is the case is still being explored. One of the characteristics of a strong friendship is the feeling of mattering to each other. In this study, researchers set out to investigate the role that this feeling of mattering plays in the link between friendship and happiness.

They specifically looked not at the quality of the friendship, or how much people actually mattered to their friends, but how much they *perceived* that they mattered to their friends. Our perception of how much we matter to our friends can be affected by the amount of attention they give to us compared with the amount of attention they give to other people and things in their lives. We may also compare our friends' behaviour with our experiences of other people in the past to form a judgement about how much we matter to them.

For the study, 196 psychology students with an average age of twenty-three were recruited from a Midwestern university in the US. In exchange for extra credit in their psychology classes, the students completed questionnaires which measured friendship quality, perceived mattering and happiness. Before answering the questions, they were provided with a definition of friendship for the purpose of the study to ensure that they weren't all thinking about different types of relationships. The definition excluded romantic partners and anyone they had any type of sexual involvement with or romantic interest in.

The results showed that the students' perceptions of how much they mattered to their three closest friends explained the link between happiness and friendship quality. The researchers cautioned we can't assume that this finding applies to people who aren't in college or other age groups. More research would be needed to explore whether the same result occurs among different sections of the population and people in different countries, but the study supports the theory that it's not how good the friendship is that matters, but how much we think we matter to our friends.

Happiness hint ☑

Find friends you think you matter to (even if really you don't).

I just asked my co-author David if my friendship mattered to him, and he said, 'What matters is your perception', with a laughing emoji – so I'm going to take that as a no! Thanks a lot, David.

Luckily for me, I do have friends I think I matter to – especially my closest friends Kieran, John and Lucy – but I also know for sure that I matter to my daughter, and that gives my life meaning and purpose.

Of course, there are plenty of things I talk to my friends about that I can't talk about with my eleven-year-old (and vice versa, as my friends don't really want to talk about space robots, or what Jaxon said to Harrison in Year 6).

I think that without close true friends in my life, I'd be a hell of a lot lonelier. The friends I have these days are kind, unsuperficial souls who treat others well. I cherish the time I get to spend with them, and if I ever come into a lot of money they'll be seeing the proceeds.

I really look forward to seeing Grandad John on a Friday (he's not my biological grandad, it's just his nickname). There's nothing like putting the kettle on and sitting down with a hot mug of tea for a chat with a mate you feel totally at ease with. Putting the world to rights and rambling about everything and nothing is one of the best things in the world.

In a way, it's up there with being in love, except being in love is generally transient and conditional, whereas friendships tend to last much longer and are less conditional. Grandad has seen me at my worst and he's still my friend, so I can relax in the knowledge that he's not going to turn his back on me if I get upset or angry.

I found this line interesting: 'Our perception of how much we matter to our friends can be affected by the amount of attention they give to us compared with the amount of attention they give to other people and things in their lives.' I've been friends with people for a generation who eventually coupled up and started to pay a lot less attention to me, which was sad and hurtful – as if I was just a placeholder for their new partner. But these things happen, and I certainly wouldn't want them to spend time with me if they'd much rather be with their partner and were counting the seconds until they could get back to them!

So maybe ask yourself: which friends matter to you, and do you think you matter to them equally? I hope so.

Reference:
Demir M., Özen A., Doğan A., Bilyk N.A., Tyrell F.A., I Matter to My Friend, Therefore I am Happy: Friendship, Mattering, and Happiness. *J Happiness Stud.* 2011;12(6):983–1005.

Having real-world friends

Research study 🗁

Title: Comparing the Happiness Effects of Real and Online
   Friends

Year: 2013

Country: Canada

As many bemoan the continuing cultural shift away from face-to-face
(or 'real-world') interactions, some researchers have suggested that
online connections might actually provide more effective ways of
building relationships, offsetting any harm to our wellbeing from the
loss of traditional friendships.

To investigate whether this is true, researchers analysed data from a
large online Canadian survey conducted in 2011. Called the 'Happiness
Monitor', and sponsored by Coca-Cola, the survey gathered data from
over five thousand Canadian residents aged 16+, from all across the
country. For this study, the researchers analysed the answers to questions
on the size of participants' social networks, their levels of happiness and
personality, as well as basic information such as age and income.

To measure happiness, the participants had been asked to imagine a
ladder with steps numbered from zero at the bottom to ten at the top
and say where they were on the ladder currently if the top of the ladder

represented their best possible life and the bottom represented their worst possible life.

After taking account of other factors which might influence happiness, such as income and stress, the results of the analysis showed that generally the more real-life friends people had, the happier they were. The authors concluded that doubling your number of friends has the same effect on happiness as a 50% increase in your income. On the other hand, the size of people's online networks was largely unrelated to how happy they were. They also found that having real-life friends appeared to be much more important for the happiness of those who weren't in a relationship compared to those who were married or living with a partner.

This study provides evidence that online friends are not as beneficial as real-world ones when it comes to happiness, although the analysis doesn't tell us for definite that one of these things is caused by the other. There's also the possibility that the link between different friendship types and happiness varies between different cultures and generations.

Happiness hint ☑

Try building more friendships in the real world and not just gaining more followers online.

Oh God, yeah – my online friendship with a lovely guy called Kieran was nice, but it became so much better when it turned into an offline friendship, when I advertised one of my gigs on Facebook and he turned up. A hot, single thirty-five-year-old sitting in the front row of one of my gigs literally *never* happens, so I got a bit flustered!

We've become close friends since, and lovers, and also have an on-off exclusive romantic relationship.

Part of the reason it's an on-off relationship is that Kieran lives with his parents 150 miles away and, for complex reasons, can't move out for ages. He also doesn't want kids. Sometimes I can deal with being in a relationship with someone in this situation, and sometimes I find it difficult. I have borderline personality disorder, so have problems with stability in relationships.

Sure, I have ten thousand Twitter followers, and among them are some truly kind people whom I've formed good online friendships with, but these are nowhere near as close as my handful of really close real-life mates who I can hug and kiss and enjoy cups of tea with.

Kieran, John and Lucy are all genuinely great people and spending time with them is the best thing in the world after spending time with my daughter.

The thing with online friendships is that you don't actually know whether those people would like you in real life. You have no idea whether you'd click as people, or endure long silences in conversation where you're tempted to claim your house is on fire so you can get to go home.

The connections are based on a shaky footing, and I often follow people based on a ten-word bio and have no idea what they're really like.

Also, I've experienced fun and enjoyable connections with people online, only for them to then unfollow me for no discernible reason, leaving me thinking, 'Well, that was unexpected – I'm not sure what happened there!' And you can't even ask them without looking a bit weird.

I can honestly say that I don't think Kieran, John or Lucy would ever unfollow me online unless we'd had a proper bust-up (which I can't see happening either). Online friendships come and go, but these are proper friendships, and I can't imagine being without any of them now.

Reference:
Helliwell J.F., Huang H., Comparing the Happiness Effects of Real and On-Line Friends. *PLoS One*. 2013;8(9):1–17.

The Happiness Interview: Derren Brown

Derren Brown is an illusionist, mentalist, artist and bestselling author. During a varied and notorious TV career, he has played Russian roulette live, convinced middle-managers to commit armed robbery, led the nation in a seance, stuck viewers at home to their sofas, successfully predicted the National Lottery, motivated a shy man to think he was landing a packed passenger plane at 30,000 feet, hypnotised a man to assassinate Stephen Fry and created a zombie apocalypse for an unsuspecting participant after seemingly ending the world. His last two bestselling books, A Little Happier: Notes for Reassurance *and* Happy: Why More or Less Everything is Absolutely Fine *(Transworld), explored changing concepts of happiness.*

What three things make you happiest?

Dinners with friends I haven't seen for a while.

A productive afternoon of writing or painting.

The rare mornings I wake up refreshed.

What three things would make you happier?

More of the above.

If my partner and I shared more similar estimations of what constituted stress.

Seeing friends more often.

What advice would you give to anyone who wants to be happy?

Firstly, ditch the goal of being happy: it can't be chased directly. Instead, seek *greater meaning*, and a robust happiness will come as a by-product. You create meaning by finding something bigger than yourself and throwing yourself into that. So pay attention to what that thing might be.

Secondly, make your peace with the fact that the world doesn't do as it's told. People will disappoint you every day, and you will fail to meet your own standards. All of this is okay. You only really need to concern yourself with how you think and act: nothing bad will happen if you decide that what the rest of the world does is fine just as it is. So, have high intentions but low expectations.

Spending time with friends

Research study 🗀

Title: Country Roads, Take Me Home . . . to My Friends:
How Intelligence, Population Density, and Friendship
Affect Modern Happiness

Year: 2016

Country: USA

Some academics have hypothesised that our level of happiness is influenced by our deep-rooted primeval instincts. They call this the 'savanna theory of happiness'. The idea is that it's not just the consequences of a particular situation or event in our contemporary lives that affects how happy or unhappy it makes us, but also the consequences it would have had for our early human ancestors on the plains of Africa. Those who subscribe to this theory believe that what would have made our ancestors happy or unhappy has the same effect on us as well. It's also suggested that the influence of these ancestral urges is greater for people with a lower level of intelligence.

Influenced by this theory, researchers from Singapore and the UK used data from the US to test out their prediction that how often we socialise with friends affects our level of happiness. Our ancestors are believed to have lived in groups of around 150, in which frequent social contact would have been necessary for survival. It's therefore assumed that experiencing less social interaction in this environment would be detrimental to happiness. The data used was collected in *National Longitudinal Study of Adolescent Health*, which involved interviews with 15,197 people aged eighteen to twenty-eight between 2001 and 2002. The participants had originally been recruited from a representative selection of US schools for another study some years earlier.

They were asked questions which measured happiness, intelligence and how often they socialised with friends in the last seven days. Once the participants' marital status had been factored in, the analysis of the data showed that more frequently socialising with friends was linked with greater happiness. It also turned out that this link was significantly stronger among the least intelligent people. Among the most intelligent people, spending more time with friends was actually linked with experiencing less happiness rather than more. The researchers hypothesised that this might be because less intelligent people have more trouble coping with the 'evolutionary novelty' of spending less time in the company of friends than their hunter-gatherer ancestors.

We can't rule out that being unhappy affected the amount of time people spent with friends rather than the other way around. Nevertheless, the findings provide some evidence to support the idea that our primitive urge to socialise has a role to play in determining how happy we are – at least for those of us who aren't especially brainy.

Happiness hint ☑

If you're not very bright, spend lots of time hanging out with your friends. If you are very bright, it's best not to overdo it.

I feel I can't win here. Either I admit to loving seeing my friends and seem like a dunce or I say I *don't* especially like seeing them and offend them in the process!

Truthfully, it's definitely the former, and I really struggled with the lack of company during the pandemic lockdowns. Though as far as intelligence goes, I'd like to point out indignantly that I'm a former champion of TV's words-and-numbers gameshow *Countdown* and also won the top prize on the puzzle-based show *BrainTeaser*!

Rather than assume I'm dim, I think we need to factor in that I'm an extremely gregarious person – a factor that's missing from the study. I'm sure your level of extraversion is as important to the findings as your level of intelligence. My lovely friend Lucy is just as intelligent as me, but is more introverted and doesn't need as much company.

I wonder if there's also an element to this study where less intelligent people are less likely to spend their time on creative pursuits such as writing books, and are more likely to spend their time watching TV. If you're working on an exciting new creative project then chances are that, even if you like your friends a lot, you might resent the distraction of spending time with them and wish you were absorbed in your project instead – whereas TV-watching can be combined with seeing your mates.

I've also met a few super-intelligent people who are a bit aloof and haughty and think they're better than everyone else, so it's unsurprising that they wouldn't enjoy socialising. Time with friends is never gonna be fun if you spend it thinking, 'God, they're thick!'

Reference:
Li N.P., Kanazawa S., Country roads, take me home . . . to my friends: How intelligence, population density, and friendship affect modern happiness. *Br J Psychol.* 2016;107(4):675–97.

Dining with company

Research study 🗁

Title: With Health and Good Food, Great Life! Gender Differences
and Happiness in Chilean Rural Older Adults

Year: 2015

Country: Chile

A group of researchers conducted a study to find out what factors determined the happiness of elderly people living in rural areas, and whether these differed between men and women.

One of the topics the researchers focused on was how satisfied people were with their food and how this related to how happy they felt overall.

The study was conducted in the Maule Region of Chile – the country's most rural area. Trained interviewers were sent out to ask 385 older people (241 women and 144 men) standard sets of questions used to measure happiness, levels of satisfaction with the food-related facets of life, and other aspects of people's quality of life. The average age of the women they spoke to was seventy-one and the average age of the men was seventy-three.

After analysing the data, the researchers found that satisfaction with diet, being independent in daily activities and feeling in good health were all linked with happiness. Men and women were equally likely to be happy; however, there were differences between the sexes in which factors were associated with happiness. In women, the results showed that how often they had dinner with someone else was related to how happy they were. The likelihood of them describing themselves as 'very happy' increased the more frequently they dined with a companion.

The analysis also showed that women were less likely to be happy if they weren't the person in the household who was responsible for buying food (although only 22% of women said they were in this category).

To what extent these findings might also apply to non-rural areas and other parts of the world isn't clear.

Happiness hint ☑

Have meals with other people more often (especially if you're an elderly woman in a rural area).

Isn't this just because the more friends there are in your life, the happier you are? When we were in the depths of lockdown and I'd barely seen anyone except my daughter for months, I felt incredibly low. I'd spend wonderful weekends with Lily, but she was often with her dad during the week, and I wasn't allowed to see anyone else, so was extremely lonely – much like everyone around the world in the same situation, I imagine.

Also, sharing food is a lovely thing. There's something magical about having dinner – the anticipation of delicious food (particularly that which you yourself have chosen), the sparkling conversation, the low lighting, the knowledge that you'll be enjoying each other's company for a good few hours. I strongly suspect these pleasures aren't confined to the Maule Region of Chile!

And I think that's a reason why I'm currently less happy than I could be: as ever, I'm on a diet, and am subsisting on protein drinks. I don't think the women in the study would have been quite as happy if they'd been dining with a companion while slurping a 130-calorie protein drink full of dried soy! The inability to share the same food with anyone is a bit miserable (I mean, theoretically I'd share my soy, but I'm not willing to inflict such a pitiful meal on my friends).

Imagine that 'celebrity dinner party' question – 'Which three people, alive or dead, would you invite to a dinner party?' – except, instead of choosing AOC, John Lennon and Malala, you choose your friends and family instead. Which of your loved ones would you cherish having dinner with most?

Reference:
Lobos G., Grunert K.G., Bustamante M., Schnettler B., With Health and Good Food, Great Life! Gender Differences and Happiness in Chilean Rural Older Adults. *Soc Indic Res*. 2016; 127(2):865–85.

Social capital

Research study 📁

Title: Searching for Happiness: The Importance of Social Capital

Year: 2013

Country: Canada

The concept of social capital is based on the idea that we acquire benefits from our social connections. These benefits can be thought of as resources, or 'capital', which accumulate as we form ties with others and build a sense of community.

Researchers used data from a large Canadian survey to look for associations between happiness and measures of social capital at an individual level. The General Social Survey on Social Engagement, 2003 collected information from almost twenty-five thousand people aged fifteen and over selected to provide a representative sample of Canada's total population. The survey included questions on a wide range of topics, including wellbeing, cultural background, social participation, political participation and education, as well as details such as age, sex and marital status.

For this study, the researchers analysed data from the survey which related to various aspects of social capital, including questions on trust in other people, trust in institutions such as the police, health care system and banks, sense of belonging, giving and receiving help from others, and participation in politics and civic society. They found that happiness was associated with some (but not all) aspects of social capital, including trust in one's family members, trust in institutions, feeling close to a greater number of relatives and having a sense of belonging to the local community.

Although the results don't prove that happiness is caused by these things, the study provides some evidence to support the idea that how much social capital people have in their lives might play a role in determining how happy they are.

Happiness hint ☑

Live in a community you feel part of, try not to be too cynical about big institutions and build trust with your relatives.

Oh my word, I have *no* social capital whatsoever! Unless we're talking about friends. Does it include friends?

The only relative except for my daughter whom I speak to with any regularity is my mum. Though I love her, as longstanding readers of my books will know, our relationship has historically been difficult. She mainly calls me so she can speak to my daughter; either that or she wants tech support from me as her phone has gone wrong. I'm not sure this is entirely what you mean by social capital! I do trust her, though; she's very reliable.

I love my nan too, but she's ninety-six, has dementia and I don't know how much she's aware of any more. Other than them, I have no relatives I'm in touch with.

I have no feelings about banks and social institutions; I'm not sure I either trust or mistrust them. They're just *there*, aren't they? I am a fan of the NHS, our wonderful healthcare service in the UK, but I also largely try to stay away from doctors and hospitals since David told me in our last book that around one hundred thousand people die each year worldwide due to healthcare mistakes and infections from medical treatment!

I don't really feel part of my community and I don't know any of my neighbours, which is pretty standard for London where I live, and big cities in general; people like to keep to themselves. I used to be a member of the Nextdoor (neighbourhood app) group for my area, but it wasn't very geared towards happiness; a typical post on the group was 'Dead cat in wheelie bin!!!! DISGUSTING!!!!'

I think perhaps I need to volunteer and join in some local community initiatives. My street is always full of litter, so maybe I'll go out with a grabby stick and a bin bag? Unless, of course, I come across a dead cat.

Reference:

Leung A., Kier C., Fung T., Fung L., Sproule R., Searching for Happiness: The Importance of Social Capital. In: Delle Fave A. (ed.), *The Exploration of Happiness*, Happiness Studies Book Series, Dordrecht: Springer; 2013:247–67.

The Happiness Interview: Jeremy Vine

Jeremy Vine is a presenter, broadcaster and journalist. He is best known as the host of his own BBC Radio 2 programme, which features news, opinions, interviews with live guests and popular music. He is famous for his direct presenting style, and exclusive reporting from war-torn areas throughout Africa. He also presents the long-running BBC quiz show Eggheads, *as well as his own daily Channel 5 current affairs show,* Jeremy Vine.

What three things make you happiest?

Doing what my dad did, which was just to sit in the garden with a book. I always said he had the house of a thousand bookmarks, because he never finished books. And not finishing a book makes me very happy! In other words, not being on a deadline and meeting a deadline, but the opposite. Having no deadline and not meeting it!

Water. I live near the Thames; I go on holiday by the sea. Water is untamed, and I think I'm pressed down by the sheer amount of stuff that humans have left their boot print on.

Music. More than ever, at the age of fifty-six, I find I'm incredibly, incredibly touched by music.

What three things would make you happier?

Doing less. When you're young and you're ambitious, you want to do everything, and as you go through life you want to do more. And there's a really important moment when you realise you want to do less, but you can't.

Being in touch with my oldest friends. I don't think I ever really tell them this, but there's five or six people I know from Durham University who I'm so close to, I could tell them anything. We've known each other for nearly forty years now, and we've been through all kinds of divorces and crises and bereavements and injuries. And the vibe when we all go out together is amazing, but we don't do it often enough.

World peace, by which I mean everyone being a bit calmer, especially on the roads when they're driving near my bicycle! And people having a plate of food on the table, and all the impossible things. The impossible dream. Because, as you get older, you do get more and more conscious that if you are privileged, your privilege in some way . . . it stands out now, it feels like an insult. And there's nothing you can do about it. And even just being born in 1965 in the UK is a huge dollop of privilege. And I'd love to see my privilege moved around a bit.

What advice would you give to anyone who wants to be happy?

Give up, forget it. Happiness is not an aim, it's a by-product. You become happy just because you weren't trying to be. People who are constantly doing a sort of mood thermostat are some of the most miserable.

Find something that you love and do it. That's so obvious, isn't it? But I've failed to become a birdwatcher. Near where I live there's the Barnes Wetlands, and I know if I went there every Saturday with a packed sandwich in tin foil, I would be happier. But I haven't managed to do it. So, if you find the thing you love, do it.

Avoid cars. Don't drive, don't get in cabs, don't get in buses. Avoid motor vehicles. They recently discovered that only the very, very most modern Teslas are immune from a very old-fashioned problem that a car has, which is that the engine burns fuel and the invisible fumes go into the driver's compartment. So if you're driving 40,000 miles a year, imagine what you're breathing in.

So my advice is: spend £200 on a bicycle. You'll never look back. That's what I did, and it changed my life.

Acts of kindness

Research study 🗁

Title: Do Unto Others or Treat Yourself? The Effects of Prosocial and Self-focused Behavior on Psychological Flourishing

Year: 2016

Country: USA

Although we often think of the pursuit of happiness as a selfish endeavour, some evidence has suggested that what really makes people happy is focusing on connecting with and supporting others. To test this out further, researchers in the US conducted a six-week experiment with 472 people aged from seventeen to sixty-seven.

They looked at the effects on mood and wellbeing of different types of behaviour by randomly assigning the participants to different groups. Some were directed to engage in acts of 'prosocial' behaviour (doing things which benefit other people) while some were directed to engage in acts of 'self-oriented' behaviour (being kind to themselves). Others were tasked with a neutral activity to provide a control group. Those in the 'prosocial' category were split further into two sub-groups. Some were asked to perform acts of kindness for other people and others were asked to do things which would benefit humanity or the wider world, rather than specific individuals.

All participants were asked to perform the same number of acts, weekly, for four weeks. At the start of the experiment, they answered questions which measured their emotions and assessed them for 'psychological flourishing' – a state of optimal mental health that goes beyond just the absence of mental illness and includes things such as high life satisfaction, self-acceptance, purpose in life and positive relations with others. After the four-week period, they were followed up a fortnight later to measure their mental wellbeing again.

The results showed that both types of prosocial behaviour improved psychological flourishing more than the self-focused or neutral activities. Those in the 'prosocial' groups experienced an increase in positive emotions and a decrease in negative emotions that wasn't seen in those who were undertaking acts of kindness directed at themselves. The data didn't show any difference in effect between the two prosocial subgroups, but in practice the acts of kindness they chose to undertake weren't as different as the researchers had intended, so this wasn't a very conclusive finding.

Overall, this study provides evidence to suggest that focusing on doing things for others may be a better strategy for improving happiness than doing things for ourselves.

Happiness hint ☑

Incorporate acts of kindness into your everyday life and treat others, not just yourself, when you need a mood boost.

You know, I've found exactly the same thing: one of my favourite things to do is perform acts of kindness for my daughter. As well as spending most of my money on her, I send her three postcards with affectionate messages each week, call her every evening, set up light boxes with a loving message on for her, buy her surprise presents such as books and stationery, and generally lavish praise and attention on her. It makes me so happy to see *her* happy.

And it's funny; chores that I wouldn't enjoy doing for myself (making my own dinner, for example) suddenly become appealing when it's about nurturing her (making her dinner and providing her with her five-a-day).

Sure, it's nice to have the occasional beauty treatment or purchase for myself, but the pleasure involved in that dissipates very quickly, especially when it comes to possessions. I guess it's a case of 'hedonic adaptation'; humans naturally adjust to having nice stuff.

But when it comes to my daughter's emotions, I don't think I will ever get tired of seeing her face light up with happiness and excitement, as it does when I buy her musical Christmas cards.

Perhaps the act of giving her presents and money also has more impact on me than doing the same for other people because, firstly, she's my daughter and I love her more than anything or anyone; and secondly, I know her so well and her reactions to gifts are absolutely genuine, whereas when I give a friend a present they tend to be less effusive, probably because they're an adult and can afford to buy most things they want themselves!

It's made me think that maybe I should perform more non-monetary acts of kindness for my friends. Which prosocial acts or acts of charity do you perform regularly, and how do they make you feel?

Reference:
Nelson S.K., Layous K., Cole S.W., Lyubomirsky S., Do unto others or treat yourself? The effects of prosocial and self-focused behavior on psychological flourishing. *Emotion*. 2016;16(6):850–61.

Sharing good news

Research study 🗁

Title: What Do You Do When Things Go Right? The Intrapersonal and Interpersonal Benefits of Sharing Positive Events

Year: 2004

Country: USA

One of the key aspects of maintaining a positive state of mental wellbeing is coping with adversity, whether that be everyday stressors or major life events, such as the death of a loved one. In times of stress, people routinely turn to others for support. We don't only share bad news with our friends and family, though – we also commonly seek out others when positive things happen in our lives. Scientists in the US conducted research to examine the impact of sharing positive news with others on people's state of mind.

They recruited 154 undergraduate students to take part in the research in exchange for extra credit towards their psychology coursework (a commonly used foolproof tactic for recruiting research participants on university campuses). The group ranged from seventeen to twenty-six years old and almost two-thirds were women. At the start of the study, they were given seven booklets to complete at the end of each day. In these booklets, participants were asked to record the most important problem or stressful event or issue of the day and the most important positive event or issue of the day. In addition, they were asked how much they'd communicated these things to others, using a five-point scale. The booklets also contained measures of mood, life satisfaction and personality. The booklets had to be handed in the next day, and any that weren't were excluded from the data when the analysis was undertaken.

The analysis took account of personality differences between the students and also the importance of the most positive and the most stressful events happening on any particular day. The results showed that when the students told someone else about the most positive event of their day, they experienced better mood and a greater sense of life satisfaction than on days when they didn't. This psychological boost went beyond that caused by the positive event itself. The benefits were even greater when the students perceived that this was met with a positive reaction, rather than a passive or negative response.

Happiness hint ☑

Get in the habit of telling others about the positive events in your daily life (preferably people who'll look happy when you do).

Ha ha. As previously stated, I used to have friends who actively seemed pissed off when things were going well for me! I stopped talking to them partly because I knew their response to my good news would be barely disguised bitterness, while they'd seem to suppress gleefulness at my bad news. And that is the *wrong way around*.

However, I do have a Taylor Swift-style squad of friends who seem happy at my good news: my Patreon supporters, who give me a little cash each month (feel free to sign up at patreon.com/ArianeSherine). In return, among other things, I send them an email full of information about the things I've done each week (entertaining stuff, not 'I went to the toilet'), and they congratulate me on the good events and commiserate on the bad. I always feel better after sending this email – I think it's very cathartic. And their joy at my happiness is lovely and genuine – you most likely wouldn't support someone financially unless you wanted the best for them.

Anyhow, this study reminds me of the old joke about the man stranded on a desert island with supermodel Cindy Crawford. They're having an amazing time, making love several times a day, but he's not satisfied with his life until he asks her to dress in *his* clothes and hat and then walk round the perimeter of the island. When she comes back into sight, he then rushes up to her and shouts, 'Dude, you won't *believe* who I'm shagging!'

There's truth to this punchline: good news is always better shared. We need people to acknowledge our successes in other ways, too; when I write a song or a piece of fiction I'm proud of, or design some stylish artwork, I send it to my friends to get their reactions, and am so pleased when they're appreciative.

Which makes me realise: I must celebrate my friends' successes more too.

Reference:
Gable S.L., Impett E.A., Reis H.T., Asher E.R., What do you do when things go right? The intrapersonal and interpersonal benefits of sharing positive events. *J Pers Soc Psychol.* 2004;87(2):228–45.

Forgiveness

Research study 🗀

Title: Forgiveness and Subjective Happiness of University Students

Year: 2017

Country: Turkey

To investigate whether a forgiving nature is linked to happiness, researchers in Turkey collected data from 828 university students.

The students answered standard sets of questions designed to measure forgiveness and their perception of their own happiness, as well as providing other personal information. The forgiveness questions measured both how forgiving the participants were towards others and how forgiving they were towards themselves.

As well as analysing the data to look for correlations between happiness and forgiveness, the researchers also wanted to find out whether the attitude of their parents was related to how forgiving the students were.

The results showed that there was a small correlation between forgiveness and happiness, with more forgiving people tending to be happier. It also turned out that the students who perceived their parents as authoritarian tended to be less forgiving than those who perceived their parents as democratic and protective. There were no significant differences between the male and female students in their levels of forgiveness and subjective happiness.

The study has some notable limitations. The correlation wasn't very big, and the data can't tell us whether there is a causal link between happiness and forgiveness or, if there is, which causes the other. Also, the study only looked at students (with an average age of twenty-one), so we can't be sure that these findings reflect what's going on in the wider general population. It does provide some evidence, though, to suggest that an attitude of forgiveness may have a role to play in happiness.

Happiness hint ☑

Being forgiving of yourself and other people *might* help make you happier (but you'll probably have to try harder to carry it off if your parents weren't the forgiving kind).

My ex-husband used to say that the contents of my grudge bank could buy out Goldman Sachs! And he was right: I don't forgive easily (except for my daughter: I'd forgive her anything).

Maybe, as the study suggests, my lack of forgiveness is due to my authoritarian parents?

But I think it's okay, especially if there's only a small correlation between forgiveness and happiness. It's not the law that you have to forgive people who have done you wrong – in fact, in evolutionary terms it makes sense not to, because if you forgive them, you might let them into your life again and give them another chance to hurt you.

Also, the number of people who are truly sorry when they say they are is small, in my experience. Most people say sorry for the pain they've caused because it's expedient for them to do so – they don't actually *believe* they were in the wrong. If I thought someone felt really bad about what they'd done and would never do it again, I'd find it far more easy to forgive them.

I can see why people who forgive others easily are happier, though – they must carry less baggage – but you can't just forgive people willy-nilly; it's not that simple. If someone's been truly horrible to you for no reason and made your life hell, you have every right to be wary and shouldn't be expected to exonerate them. It's like expecting someone to have a sudden conversion to religion to 'save their soul' when they've previously experienced the oppression religions can cause; they can't just change their personality and go, 'Very well, I'm religious now!'

Though I guess religions do have a big thing about forgiveness. Perhaps that's why I'm an atheist?

Reference:
Vural Batik M., Yilmaz Bingol T., Firinci Kodaz A., Hosoglu R., Forgiveness and Subjective Happiness of University Students. *Int J High Educ.* 2017;6(6):149–62.

The Happiness Interview: Rosie Holt

With over 250,000 Twitter followers and millions of views online, Rosie Holt's characters have been skewering the political landscape since the pandemic. Rosie is an actor and comedian and was a finalist at the Amused Moose New Comic, Leicester Square New Comedian & Bath New Act Awards. Most recently she has appeared on The Russell Howard Hour *(Sky),* Ashley Blaker: 6.5 Children *(Radio 4) and performed in the critically acclaimed two-hander* The Crown Dual *with Brendan Murphy (The Gilded Balloon/Wilton's Music Hall). She has also performed in a stage show featuring her monstrous creation, Woman Who.*

What three things make you happiest?

My friends and family.

Feeling creatively busy and fulfilled.

Sex with someone I love.

What three things would make you happier?

Being more professionally successful (sorry, I know one shouldn't measure happiness by such things, but IT WOULD).

More sex (but, in case the gods hear my cry, and this turns into some terrible 'Be careful what you wish for' scenario, to specify – GOOD sex. HAPPY sex. I've gone through periods of my life with lots of sex, and they haven't necessarily been happy periods. Am I making this too complicated?

My inability to answer these questions well makes me fear I DO NOT DESERVE happiness).

Being in love (I love being in love) with someone who loves me back. Done it before, can do it again. This specific answer could be because I am thinking about sex again.

What advice would you give to anyone who wants to be happy?

I think the more you can take a clear-eyed view and realise that what society teaches us is 'success does not equal a successful life', the happier you will be (I am still working on this one). Also realise what in your life as it stands makes you happy and capitalise on it. People make me happy, so I try to look after my friendships, as without care they can undoubtedly wilt. Food makes me happy, so I eat it. Dogs make me happy, and one day I WILL have my own.

Social media

Research study 🗀

Title: The Grass is Always Greener on My Friends' Profiles:
The Effect of Facebook Social Comparison on State Self-
esteem and Depression

Year: 2019

Country: Israel

People have always compared themselves to others in everyday life, but
the rise of social media has caused some to worry that an unhealthy
level of unrealistic comparison has now become the norm. The authors
of this study point out that what's different about online social
comparison is that it almost always involves comparing ourselves with
others who are seemingly doing better than us, rather than a mix of
people who are relatively better or worse off than ourselves. On social
media, people are much more able to edit and filter what others see of
them than they are in the real world. They primarily share the positive
aspects of their lives and present an idealised image of themselves and
their circumstances. Regularly seeing these apparently idyllic lives and
comparing them to our own can trigger negative emotions such as
shame and envy, especially for those with existing self-esteem issues.

The aim of this piece of research was to test the psychological impact
of comparing ourselves with others on Facebook – specifically the

effect on self-esteem and symptoms of depression. Participants were recruited into the study through adverts posted on social media. Eighty people took part, ranging in age from nineteen to thirty-five, all of whom were active Facebook users. Almost 70% of the participants were women. Each was given the equivalent of eight dollars in New Israeli Shekels for their time.

Initially the participants were only told that the study was looking at patterns of social network use so that their responses wouldn't be affected by knowing the specific focus of the research. They first completed questionnaires designed to measure various aspects of their psychology, including their tendency to engage in social comparison. After this, they were randomly assigned to one of two groups. One group were asked to spend fifteen minutes browsing their Facebook newsfeeds (the stream of new content and 'status updates' posted by the people they follow on the site). The other group were asked to spend the same amount of time browsing only the National Geographic Facebook page. They then filled in questionnaires designed to measure their self-esteem and levels of depression. Once this was completed, they were given the full details of what the study was looking into.

Analysis of the data collected showed that the group who browsed their Facebook newsfeed generally had lower self-esteem and higher levels of depression afterwards than those who browsed the National Geographic page (i.e. non-social content). The researchers concluded that there was evidence of a causal link between exposure to the social content and negative psychological outcomes. They also found that those who already had a higher tendency to compare themselves with others were more susceptible to the negative consequences of viewing others' Facebook updates.

The findings of this study support the theory that comparing ourselves with others through social media is damaging to our mental wellbeing, although there are some limitations to the research. The study didn't look at long-term effects, so we don't know how lasting the impact of viewing social content is. The participants were all relatively young, so we also can't be sure if older people experience the same or different effects.

Happiness hint ☑

Don't look at social media, especially if you're already prone to comparing yourself negatively to others.

There's that saying about social media, isn't there: 'Don't compare your insides with other people's outsides.' It seems like sound advice, because you never know what people are going through, even while they're putting up happy smiley Instagram posts.

I've seen stats that show that celebrities (who a lot of us follow on social media) and successful businesspeople actually have higher suicide rates than the general population, because of all the stress and pressure they're under. That's why so many also get addicted to drink and drugs. Yet it's hard to bear that in mind when you only see glossy pictures of mansions, glamorous sunshine holidays and beautiful families.

Social media is addictive – I'm on Twitter more than I should be – but we should remind ourselves that it's not a true reflection of the world. I've definitely put up cheery posts when I've been feeling glum inside, not to fool my followers but to try to distract myself from my own unhappiness. So don't be fooled by appearances: your life might actually be more fun than the lives of all the people you're envying.

Reference:
Alfasi Y., The grass is always greener on my Friends' profiles:
The effect of Facebook social comparison on state self-esteem and depression. *Pers Individ Dif.* 2019;147:111–7.

Having good sex

Research study 📁

Title: Sex and Happiness

Year: 2015

Country: China

This study used data on 3,800 randomly selected adults in China to investigate the link between good sex and happiness. The data had been collected for the China Health and Family Life Survey, conducted between 1999 and 2000 across the country among a sample of people aged twenty to sixty.

Happiness was measured by the question: 'Taken all together, how would you say things are these days – would you say that you are very happy, happy, unhappy or very unhappy?' Questions about the participants' sex lives were also included in the survey. To protect privacy and increase the likelihood of receiving honest answers, participants were brought to neutral locations away from the home to complete the survey.

The researchers used various statistical techniques to analyse the data, taking account of the health status of participants so as not to bias the results (it's assumed that people who are fit and well are generally likely to be more sexually active and fulfilled than people in very poor health). Frequency of orgasm and emotional and physical satisfaction with one's main sex partner were used to indicate the quality of sexual activity.

The main finding was that people who have better sex lives are happier. The analysis also showed that the optimum number of sex partners for maximising happiness is one. Those in exclusive long-term relationships were happier than those with multiple concurrent partners. Some variation between men and women was observed, with the physical aspects of sex having a greater impact on men's happiness and the giving and receiving of affection having a greater impact on women's happiness. Those who felt they were getting just the right amount of sex were happier than those who felt they were having too little or too much.

The results also showed that higher earners get relatively more happiness from masturbation. The researchers speculated that this might reflect their inclination to spend less time on 'leisure activities'.

Happiness hint ☑

Find one person you enjoy having sex with and don't have an affair.

'People who have better sex lives are happier.' In other news, bears defecate in wooded areas and the Bishop of Rome is Catholic.

I love having good sex, and I've never had better sex than I'm having now. I think it's to do with being comfortable with your partner – with someone who completely accepts your body and is always open to trying new things in bed, whether that's talking dirty or sex in different positions. Personally, I'm also more confident in myself now I'm forty-one, so I feel able to ask for what I want in bed rather than lying back and letting the guy call all the shots.

I'm definitely happier in an exclusive long-term relationship – each to their own, but I can't even imagine the admin and mess involved in juggling multiple relationships! I'd feel way too guilty to have an affair and don't have the slightest inclination; and who has the time for more than one boyfriend even if it's all above board?

I'm not sure why higher earners get more happiness from wanking. Perhaps they can afford to buy better sex toys? I spent £100 on my vibrator, and it was the best £100 I've ever spent. It's worked out at about 50p per orgasm so far, and the orgasms are incredible. I've never bought an orgasm but I'm sure 50p is less than the going rate!

When have you been happiest in your sex life?

Reference:
Cheng Z., Smyth R., Sex and Happiness. *J Econ Behav Organ.* 2015;112:26–32.

Avoiding pressure to have more sex

Research study 🗁

Title: Does Increased Sexual Frequency Enhance Happiness?

Year: 2015

Country: USA

Plenty of scientific studies have found that people who have sex more frequently tend to be happier. Those who have had no sexual partners in the last year are the least happy. Despite the evidence of a link between sex and happiness, scientists still didn't know whether having more sex actually made people happier or whether happiness caused people to have more sex. The link could even have been due to some third factor which was causing people to be happier and to have more sex. One theory, for example, was that being in good health might independently affect people's happiness and how much sex they have.

In this study, researchers in the US set out to establish whether having sex more frequently actually makes people happier. To do this they recruited heterosexual married couples aged thirty-five to sixty-five, split the couples into two groups randomly and asked one group to double the number of occasions when they had sexual intercourse. Couples who had sexual problems in their relationship or experienced physical discomfort during intercourse were excluded. People with certain health problems, such as high blood pressure, and those who had sex less than once a month or more than three times a week were also kept out of the study.

Before starting the experiment, participants completed questionnaires to assess their mental and physical wellbeing, happiness and libido. They were then asked daily questions using standard measures on how they were feeling, how much they wanted sex, whether they'd had sex and whether it gave them an orgasm.

When they analysed the results, the researchers found that those who'd been induced to have more sex were less happy than those who hadn't. How much more sex the couples had didn't seem to determine how much more unhappy they were. Rather, it seemed that it was the act itself of instructing people to have more sex that made them want sex less, enjoy it less and feel less happy.

The experiment failed to establish the effect on happiness of having more sex under normal circumstances, but instead showed that a burden of expectation to increase sexual frequency can make people feel worse generally and reduce the pleasure they get from sex.

Happiness hint ☑

Forcing yourself to have more sex just to be happier might make you unhappier.

I'm nearly always in the mood for sex, but I can also understand that sex is only fun and hot if you actively feel turned on and want to do it. I remember nine months (ironically) of trying (and failing) to get pregnant with my then-husband. Sex suddenly became less about physical pleasure, and more about getting up the duff – shouting 'I'm ovulating, let's do it quickly!' doesn't tend to lend itself to sizzling rutting.

I'm pretty sure pressure of any kind is anathema to sexual arousal. You're meant to be thinking, 'Fuck, yeah, I want to rip your clothes off and do all kinds of kinky things to your body!' not, 'Fuck, I'm old and my eggs are shrivelling up!' or, 'Fuck, I'm so bored of sex under duress!'

And having sex when you don't physically want to, even in a loving relationship, can have adverse consequences for both sexes: for women, it can be painful, even with lube, and lead to lack of orgasms; for men, it can mean embarrassment if they can't sustain an erection or come.

In our last book *How to Live to 100*, we said that you should try to have sex twice a week if possible to maximise your life expectancy. However, having more sex than this was actually less effective at extending your life than having sex twice, possibly because sex twice a week is the upper limit for most long-term couples and more than this might mean having sex through gritted teeth.

As a friend of mine in a long-term relationship moaned recently, 'Twice a WEEK? That's a lot, Ariane – we've been together for *ten years!*'

What would your optimum frequency be?

Reference:
Loewenstein G., Krishnamurti T., Kopsic J., McDonald D., Does Increased Sexual Frequency Enhance Happiness? *J Econ Behav Organ.* 2015;116:206–18.

The Happiness Interview: Mhairi McFarlane

Mhairi McFarlane is the author of seven romantic comedies, all published by HarperCollins, and her eighth, Mad About You, *is out now. Her sixth novel,* If I Never Met You, *is under option for a screen adaptation. She lives in Nottingham with a man and a cat, and spends an inordinate amount of time pissing about and chatting on social media, claiming she is 'soaking up inspiration' for her work. Her hobby is reading restaurant menus online, and she has no intention of ever going skiing.*

What three things make you happiest?

Writing,

Time with friends, hopefully involving food and wine and no topic censorship.

Anticipating a curry and having the curry, I enjoy it so much that the former is almost as good as the latter.

What three things would make you happier?

Everyone being nicer on social media (probably me included).

More exercise (pretty much never fails as a good mood pill).

The surprise announcement that David Fincher is making three more series of his period-piece psychological crime thriller *Mindhunter*.

The Happiness Interview: Mhairi McFarlane

What advice would you give to anyone who wants to be happy?

'Happy' is a fraught and complicated word, in my opinion, as we use it to mean different things. It all too often stands as code for 'has life arranged conventionally, and correctly. Has all the big-ticket ingredients for happiness in the eyes of others.' Career, money, a photogenic family, good looks, popularity, good health. You only need to see how mystifying and fascinating people find it that a glamorous celebrity could ever be miserable to understand that we think happiness = having enviable things, and attributes.

Happiness isn't actually anything to do with how your life looks from the outside, or what would make someone else happy – it's really about a state of quiet, appreciative contentment in your own existence. To quote Warren Zevon, it's in enjoying every sandwich. I'm really wary of sounding like a Live Laugh Love decal and trying to avoid the word 'gratitude', but in the twenty-first century, it's so easy to see happiness as something that will arrive when 'X' does. And of course, when you make happiness about achievements, it's a forever moving target. And most of the things we want to happen come with their own challenges and complications. The secret of all happy people I know is their valuing what they already have, and pausing to enjoy the moment.

This is going to sound insufferably twee, but bear with me – this week, I opened a window in the morning and the fresh air smelled incredible. I am usually a winter hater, yet it was foggy, smoky and crisp, in a really nice way. The thought I could get dressed and go out into that air made me, for a moment, really happy. (Everyone reading: 'Is this bitch drunk?')

Swinging

Research study 🗀

Title: Swinging High or Low? Measuring Self-esteem in Swingers

Year: 2018

Country: USA

There's plenty of evidence that happiness is linked with self-esteem, so any activity which gives it a boost could be valuable in helping people become happier. Some research has suggested a belief among swinging couples that the practice increases their self-esteem. In this study, researchers set out to explore whether people involved in a consensually non-monogamous relationship really do have higher self-esteem than the general population.

To do this, they teamed up with a local swingers' club and got permission to set up a table with questionnaires at one of their events. Forty-one swingers approached the table and volunteered to complete the questionnaire. There were nineteen men and twenty-two women, with an average age of forty-five. Most of the participants were married. The questionnaire gathered data on basic characteristics, such as age, sex and religion, and measured self-esteem using a recognised scale. It also measured the participants' general tendency to give socially desirable or favourable responses, to give some insight into how likely they were to give what they thought were the 'right' answers, rather than truthful ones. Due to the stigma surrounding swinging, the researchers were concerned this may be an issue, but it turned out not to be.

When analysing the results, they compared them with existing data from previous surveys of the general population. Their analysis revealed that, generally, male swingers have higher self-esteem than the norm, but female swingers' self-esteem is not significantly different from that of others.

The researchers theorised that some aspects of the swinging lifestyle may help men to feel better about themselves, including the higher number of sexual partners and the greater opportunities to reproduce (both of which are known to be linked to male self-esteem). The data in this study are only from a single point in time, however, and don't prove that men's self-esteem increases after they've begun swinging. Another limitation of the analysis is that the general population data used for comparison didn't exclude swingers, so doesn't strictly allow for a swingers vs non-swingers comparison. The researchers also pointed out that participants may have struggled to concentrate on their answers because the questionnaires were completed in a dimly lit part of the club, alcohol was being served and loud dance music was playing.

Happiness hint ☑

If you're a man, consider becoming a swinger.

The thing is, I'm not sure swinging is really a matter of choice. Personally, I need an emotional connection with someone to feel sexually attracted to them, and I don't think you get that by putting your car keys in a bowl!

And even if I did feel emotionally connected to two men and they were both open to having sex with me, I'd feel far too jealous if they were shagging other women. The whole thing is way too fraught with landmines for my liking.

And yes, I'm female, but I know men that feel the same way, so it's not just a female thing. I could be wrong, but I genuinely don't think most blokes want to be swingers – aside from anything else, it's too emotionally complicated.

Most people just want an easy, happy, safe monogamous relationship. They want to feel loved, needed and cherished, and I don't think swinging can give you that.

Reference:
Ruzansky A.S., Harrison M.A., Swinging high or low? Measuring self-esteem in swingers. *Soc Sci J.* 2019;56(1):30–37.

Pornography

Research study 🗁

Title: Is the Link Between Pornography Use and Relational
      Happiness Really More About Masturbation?
      Results From Two National Surveys

Year: 2020

Country: USA

Scientists have known for a while that people who use pornography tend to experience poorer quality romantic relationships and feel less happy in them. In this study, researchers set out to discover whether this link could be explained by a third factor – masturbation.

They speculated that because people typically masturbate while watching pornography, the masturbation may have more to do with how happy people felt in their romantic relationships than viewing pornography in itself.

The researchers used existing data on 12,083 adults from two national surveys – the 2012 New Family Structures Study and the 2014 Relationships in America Survey. Both surveys asked questions which measured participants' happiness with their current relationships, their pornography viewing frequency and their masturbation habits. Data from the surveys on other factors which could muddy the waters, such as religious beliefs, income, depression and frequency of having sex, were also taken from the surveys and factored into the analysis.

The data showed an average pornography usage of once a month or less. Around a fifth of the participants stated that they never masturbated. The analysis suggested that those who masturbated more frequently were generally less happy in their romantic relationships. Once masturbation habits were taken into account, the data showed no evidence that pornography has a negative effect on happiness. In contrast with previous research, it even suggested that, for men, viewing pornography might be linked with being happier with one's relationship.

The researchers concluded that, because data on the participants' sex lives with their partners was taken into account in the analysis, it was unlikely that more frequent masturbation simply reflected a dissatisfaction with their sexual relationship that was also making the participants unhappy. They theorised instead that regular masturbation may itself detract from the relationship, although this wasn't proven definitively by the study.

Happiness hint ☑

If you're in a relationship, don't masturbate a lot (but if you're a man you might want to watch some porn).

It doesn't say whether the people in this study were living together. I'm in a long-distance relationship, and my bloke Kieran and I only see each other a couple of times a month, so we're not going to hold off on wanking! I don't think wanking is a sign that we're not happy with our sexual relationship at all, far from it – if we lived together we probably wouldn't do much solo sexual activity.

But as we're apart so much, we need to release our sexual frustration. However, we do involve each other – we exchange sexy photos and videos and effectively use them as porn, it's just that it's porn of each other rather than of strangers. And we talk dirty to each other a lot and describe what we want to do to each other the next time we're together.

I've never felt comfortable sending sexy photos or videos to anyone before, but Kieran's so appreciative of my body and finds me so sexy that I'm happy to send him naked selfies, safe in the knowledge that he isn't going to go, 'Ugh!' Also, I completely trust that he'll never show my photos or videos to anyone.

And even if they do leak someday, I'm sure the world isn't gonna be *that* interested in my tits and fanny, because the internet's full of millions of the things!

I genuinely think watching porn makes you feel a bit grubby, though. And I haven't watched any for six years after reading a study that showed that women in porn largely have traumatic backgrounds. I thought, 'That could be me.'

So I just use my imagination these days, which I find hotter anyway.

Reference:
Perry S.L., Is the Link Between Pornography Use and Relational Happiness Really More About Masturbation? Results From Two National Surveys. *J Sex Res.* 2020;57(1):64–76.

Non-committal relationships

Research study 📁

Title: Together is Better: Higher Committed Relationships Increase
Life Satisfaction and Reduce Loneliness

Year: 2019

Country: Germany

The authors of this study noted that the proportion of people who
were in couples went down between 2004 and 2014, despite the
increasing availability of online dating platforms and increasing social
acceptance of their use. Academics have theorised that the increased
opportunity to meet potential partners, ironically, may have
undermined the formation of stable and committed romantic
relationships. The suggestion is that the seemingly endless availability
of alternative potential suitors that dating platforms provide reduces
the inclination to commit to one partner – both for fear of missing out
on a better alternative and because it is now easier to maintain an
active sex life without having a stable partner.

The researchers set out to explore the association between people's
relationship status and level of happiness – specifically how lonely they
feel and how satisfied they are with their lives. The study had a
particular focus on the concept of 'mingles' – a term for people who
are neither single nor in a committed romantic relationship. Mingles

are in a monogamous intimate relationship with another person in private but do not commit to that person and in public identify themselves as single.

The participants in the study were 764 students at a German university, ranging from seventeen to fifty-nine years old, who had signed up to take part in different research projects. They completed an online questionnaire which collected data on age, gender and level of education, as well as current relationship status and the duration of this status. Questions were also asked which measured how satisfied the participants were with their lives, their level of loneliness, the extent to which they felt committed to their current partner and their level of commitment to that partner. One year prior to this study being undertaken, 244 of the participants had also completed a survey which gathered data on relationship status, life satisfaction and loneliness, allowing the researchers to look at how these things had changed over time for these individuals.

The study showed that adults in committed relationships were more satisfied with their lives and less lonely than mingles and singles, with singles faring worst of the three groups. The analysis also suggested that women tend to feel that their needs are not met in relationships with low commitment, whereas this was not the case for men. When they looked at the data collected a year earlier, the researchers also discovered that those who shifted into a more committed form of relationship generally became less lonely and felt more satisfied with their lives than they had before.

Happiness hint ☑

If you're single, get into a relationship, even if you can't commit. If you're in a non-committal relationship, switch to one that's committal.

Well, to start with, 'mingles' makes me think of 'mingers', which isn't very appealing. And their behaviour isn't appealing either – who wants a partner who refuses to commit to you and tells everyone they're single?

I imagine that some of these people's unhappiness is probably based on the fact that their long-suffering partner keeps starting steaming rows with them about their commitment phobia!

But yeah, who *wouldn't* feel happier in a relationship that's on a secure footing? I mean, if you like someone enough to want to spend time with them and allow bits of them into your body or vice versa, surely you want a stronger relationship than 'meh, we're not a couple'? I'd find it positively insulting if someone was boffing me then pretending I meant nothing to them (and worse still if I *actually* meant nothing to them!).

I see ENM in loads of profiles on dating apps, though – apparently it stands for 'ethically non-monogamous' and basically means shagging around but letting everyone know you're shagging around (that's the ethical bit). I suppose if everyone's cool with it and it doesn't harm anyone, who am I to be an old grandma nagging people about morality?

All I'm saying is, it's not very romantic and it doesn't surprise me that being in a committed relationship makes people happier than being in a non-committal relationship. It may be old-fashioned, but that doesn't mean it's not for the best.

Reference:
Bucher A., Neubauer A.B., Voss A., Oetzbach C., Together is Better: Higher Committed Relationships Increase Life Satisfaction and Reduce Loneliness. *J Happiness Stud.* 2019;20:2445–69.

The Happiness Interview: Femi Oluwole

Femi Oluwole is a political activist and anti-Brexit campaigner. He is the co-founder of the pro-European Union advocacy group Our Future Our Choice, regularly appears on television and radio, and has written for the Guardian, *the* Independent *and the* Metro.

What three things make you happiest?

Feeling useful: knowing that my best skills are being used to help others. Almost makes the childhood trauma feel worth it, like, at least someone else is suffering less because of what I went through.

Intellectual connection with someone on a niche topic, e.g. Buffy.

Adrenalin sports.

What three things would make you happier?

A relationship with someone who I could share the above three things with.

A dog.

More career success.

What advice would you give to anyone who wants to be happy?

Be careful whose eyes you judge yourself through. It could be your parents'. Especially your partner's. They will have their own flaws. Figure out what values you think make someone a good person. And as long as you know you're doing your best to do that, stop attacking yourself.

Couple similarity

Research study 🗁

Title: Couple Similarity and Marital Satisfaction:
Are Similar Spouses Happier?

Year: 2006

Country: Israel

A key question for academics interested in human relationships is whether romantic partners who are similar to each other have better quality relationships and feel happier than those who have little in common.

Israeli researchers set out to answer this by analysing data on married couples who were part of a larger piece of research on work and family. They looked at a sample of 248 heterosexual Jewish Israeli married couples who had been recruited on to the study through day-care centres and community child-health facilities. The participants ranged in age from twenty to fifty-nine and all of the couples had at least one child. Roughly three-quarters had some college-level education. The couples were visited in their homes by researchers and asked to fill in comprehensive questionnaires which took them around an hour to complete.

The data used in this study was gathered through questions designed to measure personality traits, attitudes to the roles of husbands and wives in the family, marital satisfaction and mood over the previous two weeks, as well as basic characteristics such as age, education and how religious someone is.

The analysis of the data showed that people who were more similar to their partners were generally more satisfied with their marriages and experienced lower levels of negative feelings. Similarities in personality and shared values were shown to be particularly important. Similarities between partners in how religious they were appeared to be less critical.

While similarity within married couples was found to be clearly related to experiencing fewer negative feelings, this wasn't the case for positive feelings. In other words, couples with higher similarity were less likely to experience bad feelings rather than being more likely to experience good feelings. The researchers suggested that this may reflect a greater level of conflict between couples who are poorly matched.

As the data was all collected from people who were straight and with young children, we can't say whether similar patterns apply among couples who don't fit into this category. The study also didn't prove that similarity between partners caused them to feel better than more dissimilar couples, or whether happy people in happy relationships tend to develop more common ground with their partners over time. The researchers noted, however, that other studies have tended to show that partners with a high level of similarity tend to start off similar rather than becoming that way once they have become a couple. This would provide some evidence to suggest that being happier with your marriage and feeling less negative might be partly caused by being similar to your partner.

Happiness hint ☑

Marry someone similar to yourself.

Couple similarity

Ha ha, 'marry someone similar to yourself'?! I'm a half-Parsi half-American mixed-race atheist Londoner with a Zoroastrian mum, a Unitarian Universalist dad and a weird German half-brother. I also have enough mental health disorders to fill a page of A3, including BPD, OCD and GAD, so the chances of me meeting someone similar are pretty remote.

But okay, I know what you mean. I've dated a lot of guys in the media and there's always a kind of 'ahhh' of compatibility when you realise you both completely understand each other. I think it's important to have similar political and religious views, too, and similar interests. I'm pretty averse to strenuous exercise so I don't think I'd match well with anyone who was obsessed with running.

My last relationship was crap in pretty much every way, but the final time I saw my ex – the first and only time I visited his house – I realised how utterly incompatible we were. I don't watch much telly, but all he wanted to do was watch QVC and *Come Dine with Me*!

He literally sat in front of the telly staring at it all evening and criticising the people on the screen. I hope he finds another QVC-obsessive to spend his life with, though it's probably remiss of me to inflict him on them.

Kieran and I don't have a whole lot in common, unfortunately. Still, unlike several of my exes, he's a wonderful person who always acts with kindness. He's also super-smart, and built an Enigma machine and got it to decode the message 'I LOVE YOU' for me.

Which is so romantic, I think I can overlook the fact that he loves Warhammer and is into historical re-enactment.

Reference:
Gaunt R., Couple similarity and marital satisfaction: Are similar spouses happier? *J Pers.* 2006;74(5):1401–20.

Dividing up the housework

Research study 📁

Title: Perceived Housework Equity, Marital Happiness, and Divorce in Dual-earner Households

Year: 2003

Country: USA

In this study, researchers chose to investigate whether happiness among married people is related to whether they think that their spouses do a fair share of the housework. They also looked at whether perceptions of fairness in the housework split were linked to subsequent divorce.

The study focused on marriages in which both spouses were earning, rather than 'traditional' marriages in which the wife stays at home to do the chores and look after the children. This was because the researchers felt that dual-earner marriages would be more prone to conflict related to housework. They used data which had already been collected from a nationally representative sample of the US population for a study which looked at marital instability between 1980 and 1988. Over two thousand people took part in the original study, but for this analysis the researchers used only the data collected from the 779 participants who were in dual-earner marriages in 1980. By 1988, when the final round of data was collected, 14% of this sample had got divorced.

Participants had been asked about how happy they were in their marriages, how much of the housework they did and whether they thought they did more than their fair share. Answers about other factors which have been shown to be related to marital happiness and divorce (including race, education, income and the presence of children) were also taken into account in the analysis.

The results showed that both husbands and wives tended to be less happy in the marriage if they perceived themselves to be doing an unfair amount of the housework. This perception of unfairness was only associated with a higher chance of divorce among women, however. There was no significant relationship between the husbands' feelings of unfairness and divorce after eight years.

Happiness hint ☑

Unless staying home to take care of the house is your thing, only marry someone who will do their fair share of the chores.

Women are usually the ones who petition for divorce, though, aren't we? I think we're responsible for initiating about two-thirds of divorces, my own included.

I remember yelling at the end of my marriage, 'You never mop the floor' and him going, 'Of *course* I do!' and me going, 'Well, you can't be mopping it very well then because it's still dirty!' My ex was meant to be doing the housework because he didn't go out to work.

I think any significant asymmetry between how much you're giving in a marriage and how much you're getting back will cause it to crumble.

I grew up in a traditional household where my dad was the main breadwinner and my mum stayed home to bring up the kids for twelve years. It was far from a happy home, but I liked the traditional aspects, because they were set in stone and were one of the few things I could rely on in my parents' turbulent marriage.

I wanted my marriage to be equal at the very least in terms of our earnings – and it wasn't. If I ever get married again, we're going to have to have a serious talk about expectations beforehand.

But to be honest, I like living by myself. At least if something isn't clean, I only have myself to blame. And no one else is going to pull me up on it.

Reference:

Frisco M.L., Williams K., Perceived housework equity, marital happiness, and divorce in dual-earner households.
J Fam Issues. 2003;24(1):51–73.

Marriage

Research study 📂

Title: Revisiting the Relationship Between Marriage and
     Wellbeing: Does Marriage Quality Matter?

Year: 2014

Country: USA, UK, Germany

Lots of research has been done which supports the theory that marriage generally has a positive effect on wellbeing. In this study, Australian scientists used data from the US, the UK and Germany to reassess the relationship between marriage and happiness and investigate the importance of marriage quality in the relationship between the two.

They analysed data which had already been collected in large population surveys in the three countries, all of which included questions designed to measure people's perceptions of their own levels of happiness and satisfaction with their lives, as well as the quality of their marriages. The US General Social Survey is a nationally representative survey of adults conducted regularly since 1972. The British Household Panel Survey began in 1991 and follows the same individuals from thousands of households over a period of years. The German Socio-Economic Panel is similar in nature and has been running since 1984.

Analysis of the data from these surveys showed that in all three countries those who were married were generally happier than those who were unmarried. They were also less likely to score in the 'least happy' category. The results suggested that being married makes people around 10% happier in the US and the UK, and around 7.5% happier in Germany.

In addition, those who assessed the quality of their marriages as poor were generally unhappy and much less happy than those who were unmarried. Those who reported their marriage quality as good, on the other hand, turned out to be even happier than expected based on the findings of previous research studies on the topic. It also turned out that the relationship between the quality of the marriage and happiness differed between the sexes. Women's happiness was much more affected by marriage quality than men's.

Another interesting finding of the study was that people who were happier were more likely to stay single rather than becoming unhappily married.

Happiness hint ☑

Get yourself into a good quality marriage. If you're unhappy and single, don't throw yourself into a poor quality marriage expecting it to make you happier.

It's a bit of a gamble then, isn't it? I mean, for the best odds, you can either get married and hope you're going to be one of the lucky ones who find themselves in a happy marriage, or stay single and be certain *not* to get into an unhappy marriage.

Having been in three abusive relationships, I'm extremely wary. I think I'd need to live with someone for over a year, with no erratic behaviour on their part whatsoever, in order to trust them enough to marry them.

Marriage

I was married for a year in 2017–2018, and though the marriage wasn't abusive, I was stressed and unhappy for most of it, because I knew that it had been a mistake.

I knew that he didn't love me, and I also knew that I didn't love him, at least not in the way I should have. After we tied the knot I felt nothing – no semblance of the giddy elation you'd hope for. And that was sad for both of us. I'm amazed the marriage lasted a year, to be honest, so I'm in no hurry to get hitched again.

But never say never.

Reference:
Chapman B., Guven C., Revisiting the Relationship Between Marriage and Wellbeing: Does Marriage Quality Matter? *J Happiness Stud.* 2016;17(2):533–51.

The Happiness Interview: Stewart Lee

Stewart Lee is one of the UK's leading comedians. He began stand-up in 1988 at the age of twenty, and won the Hackney Empire New Act of the Year Award in 1990. In 2001 he co-wrote the libretto for Richard Thomas's Jerry Springer: The Opera, *which went on to win four Olivier awards. In 2020, he teamed up with the band Asian Dub Foundation for the single 'Comin' Over Here', using a stand-up routine from his BAFTA award-winning BBC show* Stewart Lee's Comedy Vehicle. *In the same year, he wrote the documentary film* King Rocker *about the singer Robert Lloyd and the band The Nightingales, which premiered on Sky Arts in 2021.*

What three things make you happiest?

My children – I don't think my life would have any purpose without them.

A nice prehistoric stone circle or burial chamber, viewed in a lovely setting after a good walk, while drinking a flask of black tea, on a crisp clear day with a bright blue sky.

Watching otters passing stones from one paw to the other – I could do that for days.

What three things would make you happier?

Lose weight so I could get up mountains better.

Sleep more so I wasn't so ragged and anxious.

Not have constant tinnitus screaming in my brain like a choir of insane harpies.

What advice would you give to anyone who wants to be happy?

I don't know, Ariane; we're all different. I don't think there's a one-size-fits-all answer. No idea.

Not having children

Research study 📂

Title: Parenthood and Happiness: A Review of Folk Theories
Versus Empirical Evidence

Year: 2012

Country: Various

The author of this paper brought together evidence from other published academic studies relating to two questions: whether the belief that having children makes us happier is as common as we tend to think it is, and whether having children actually makes us happier in reality.

The evidence suggested that the belief that parenthood increases happiness is widely held. Studies show that 90–95% of young people around the world plan to have children, with 42% in Britain rating the importance of having children as 10/10. Fear of loneliness and depression in old age has been found to be a strong reason for having children and a very small proportion of the population intentionally remains childless through adulthood. In the US and Australia, around half of men and women think a marriage without children is not fully complete.

Surveys show that how commonly people agree with the statement 'You cannot really be happy without having children' varies considerably between countries. Only 5% agreed in the Netherlands, compared with 56% in Hungary, for example. There's a much greater level of agreement though that 'Watching children grow up is life's greatest joy'. Around the world, roughly 80–90% of people have been found to agree with this statement. British survey data showed that this proportion was notably lower among those with parenting responsibility, however.

The author couldn't find much evidence that childless adults go on to regret not being parents. Interview-based studies showed that both parents and people without children cite a range of advantages to being childless, such as greater freedom, less stress, and fewer worries and financial concerns.

Research findings from a range of countries indicate that people are generally happier without having children, but it's a complex picture. Both men and women tend to become less satisfied with their lives after the birth of their first child, but mostly get back to their previous level of happiness after the first four or five years.

There's plenty of variation between countries, though, with a lot of factors influencing the effect of parenthood on happiness, such as levels of state-based support for young families and gender equality in work. The negative impact of having children is generally greater on the people who face the greatest challenges, such as single parents and those who are financially less well off.

In countries with limited welfare systems, the negative effect on happiness of parenting young children is reversed in later life. In countries with strong welfare systems and less reliance on families to take care of the elderly, though, there's no evidence of an old-age happiness boost from being a parent.

Happiness hint ☑

Don't have children unless you'll need them to take care of you in your old age.

I'm sorry, but I'm calling bullshit on 'people are generally happier not having children'! Having my daughter Lily is genuinely the best decision I ever made, and it's why I can't regret anything about my past, as all the childhood trauma, abusive relationships and bad decisions led me to her.

Lily is kind, caring, cheeky, hilarious, smart, sassy and my whole reason for being. She's the reason I'm getting into shape, losing half my body weight so I can be healthy and stick around for her for longer; she's the reason I'm working to fulfil my dream of being a pop star, because I want to show her that she can fulfil her own dreams if she works hard enough, practises her guitar and singing and is determined and tenacious.

I'm grateful for her every minute of every day and my love for her is infinite and all-encompassing (though she tells me, 'You only love me because I'm your daughter!').

I think if children make you less happy, it's probably just because you worry about them all the time because they're so precious. Having a toddler is particularly stressful as they're so curious and you can't reason with them very well yet, so you're constantly having to stop them drinking bleach or pulling shelves down on their head.

Yes, the pre-school years are difficult – battling sleep deprivation, soothing endless crying and cleaning up explosive green poos aren't on anyone's ideal to-do list.

But I think the unconditional bond between a parent and child is the strongest emotion you can experience, much more so than other family relationships, and more so than friendships or romantic relationships too, especially as the latter are so conditional. There's no one but my daughter I'd willingly die for in a heartbeat so they could live, no one else whose life I'm determined to make truly wonderful and magical.

That said, I don't look after my daughter all the time, so I get plenty of time for myself – so perhaps that's the best of both worlds? I get to create music, writing and art during the weekdays in term time, and spend all my weekends and holidays with my daughter. I feel very lucky.

But I appreciate not everyone can structure their life like this, and I'm certainly not suggesting all couples with children split up!

Reference:

Hansen T., Parenthood and Happiness: A Review of Folk Theories Versus Empirical Evidence. *Soc Indic Res*. 2012;108:29–64.

Spending time with grandchildren

Research study 🗁

Title: The Association between Grandparental Investment and Grandparents' Happiness in Finland

Year: 2016

Country: Finland

This study explored the common perception that having grandchildren when we get older brings happiness. Researchers looked at whether those who have grandchildren are happier than those who don't and whether the level of time grandparents invest in their grandchildren is related to the level of happiness they experience.

The researchers used data from a long-running survey in Finland which regularly collects information from a nationally representative sample of baby-boomers born between 1945 and 1950. The data collected in 2012, gathered from over two thousand respondents aged around sixty-five, was analysed for this study. It included a measure of current happiness and questions on whether they had grandchildren and, if so, how frequently they had contact with them.

In the analysis, the researchers factored in their responses to other questions related to things which are known to be separately linked to happiness, such as marital status, financial circumstances and the number of emotionally close friends or relatives.

The results showed that, overall, simply being a grandparent wasn't related to happiness once these other factors had been taken into account. They did, however, find that among maternal grandmothers higher levels of contact with grandchildren were associated with higher levels of happiness. This association couldn't be explained by any of the other factors included in the analysis.

The study doesn't prove that contact with grandchildren causes higher level of happiness, rather than the other way around, and it also doesn't tell us how long the effect lasts if there is one, but it provides some evidence to suggest that maternal grandmothers might stand to benefit from throwing themselves into the role.

Happiness hint ☑

Frequently volunteer to babysit if you're a woman with a daughter who has kids.

I cannot wait to be a grandmother! Though I'm hoping it won't happen for at least fifteen years.

My daughter says she doesn't want kids, but she's only eleven so I'm not setting too much store by that. She says boys are 'yuk', 'stupid' and 'disgusting' (and she definitely has a point there), so it's unsurprising that she isn't keen on coupling up with one and starting a family.

However, I'm hoping she'll eventually change her mind. She does say she might adopt a baby alone, which would be just as good if not better, because I wouldn't have to worry about birth complications (her heart rate dropped in the womb while I was giving birth to her and I had to have an emergency caesarean, so I'd be very nervous about her giving birth).

Being a grandma would allow me to do all my favourite bits of motherhood (spoiling children, buying them lots of presents and cuddling them) without all the anxiety involved in caring for them full-time. It would also mean I could see my daughter more, which would make me very happy.

It's really interesting, though, that grandads and paternal grandmothers didn't experience a happiness boost. I'd like to come up with a revelatory reason, but I can't. When it comes to my dotage, I'm just counting my lucky stars that I'm the mum of a girl.

Reference:
Danielsbacka M., Tanskanen A.O., The association between grandparental investment and grandparents' happiness in Finland. *Pers Relatsh.* 2016;23(4):787–800.

Owning a pet

Research study 🗁

Title: Pets and Happiness: Examining the Association between Pet Ownership and Wellbeing

Year: 2016

Country: USA

Academic research has shown positive links between pet ownership and physical health, including better survival rates following a heart attack and lower blood pressure. The evidence regarding beneficial effects on mental health, however, has been mixed. In this study, the researchers wanted to see whether owning a pet is associated with positive aspects of mental wellbeing, such as happiness.

They collected data on pet ownership and happiness from 263 American adults using an online survey. There was a roughly equal split of men and women, with participants ranging in age from nineteen to sixty-eight. They were each paid three dollars to complete a set of questionnaires which used standard measures to assess their wellbeing, as well as personality traits, such as extraversion and agreeableness.

The results of the survey showed that people who owned a pet tended to be more satisfied with their lives than those who didn't. There was no difference between the two groups on other wellbeing and personality measures. Dog owners scored better than cat owners on all aspects of wellbeing, although differences in personality traits may have accounted for this finding.

Happiness hint ☑

Get a pet if you don't already have one. It might make you feel more satisfied with your life, and even if it doesn't, it might help if you have a heart attack.

Oh dear, I hope my daughter doesn't read this. She's always on at me to get a dog. I told her that dogs cost money and that I'd rather spend the money on her. She said, 'Great, give me the money and I'll spend it on a dog!'

I did think seriously about getting her a dog, but I go away on tour too much for it to be practical. I also have a home alarm system and the dog would continually trip the sensors! And dogs need walking, and it rains a third of the time, and I don't fancy walking in the rain.

There's a third option we've exercised: borrowmydoggy.com, where you pay a tenner a year to walk other people's dogs. We now walk a lovely affectionate Pomeranian once a month, and I thoroughly enjoy the experience, possibly because I'm a pom-Iranian myself.

However, despite my daughter's promises that she'll look after our dog if we get one, she always bellows, 'MUUUM! She's done a POO!' and I'm expected to pick up the stinking droppings. This takes down my happiness levels somewhat, especially as the dog is extremely fluffy and most of the poo tends to collect in her straggly bum fur, so you can smell her excrement for miles.

If you don't fancy Borrow My Doggy, I suppose you could become a dogwalker and actually get paid for it instead, but you might be asked to walk dangerous dogs.

Which reminds me: my daughter always used to go up to potentially dangerous dogs in the street as a toddler – the most snarling, vicious pit bulls and Alsatians – and go, 'Here, doggy doggy; nice doggy doggy!', stroke them roughly and pull their tails.

And I'd cringe in fear, thinking, 'This is a news story waiting to happen' – but thankfully it was all fine. One of the dogs snapped at her once, but it doesn't seem to have dimmed her enthusiasm for getting a dog.

I can see why dogs make you feel happier, especially the friendly, affectionate, sweet-natured and lovable ones, but it's just not sensible for a lot of people to get one, including me. So I've told my daughter we can get a cat instead!

Reference:
Bao K.J., Schreer G., Pets and Happiness: Examining the Association between Pet Ownership and Wellbeing. *Anthrozoos*. 2016;29(2): 283–96.

The Happiness Interview: Gordon Burns

Gordon Burns made his name nationally when he presented and scripted the popular ITV quiz show The Krypton Factor, *which ran for eighteen years in a peak-time slot and achieved audiences of up to eighteen million people. He then presented the BBC's nightly news programme* North West Tonight *for fifteen years, winning the Royal Television Society's Best News Presenter award five times and the coveted BBC Ruby Television Award for the best regional news presenter in the UK.*

What three things make you happiest?

What if what makes me happiest is not giving you an interview for your book?!

My three things are:

Waking up in the morning as it's by no means guaranteed at my ripe old age! [Gordon is eighty.]

Being known by all four of my fabulous grandchildren as 'silly-old-papa'.

Beating Australia in an Ashes Test Match.

What three things would make you happier?

Waking up in the morning this day next year and any day thereafter.

Knowing Ariane Sherine has become such a huge success she doesn't have to ask me boring questions like these any more.

Managing to actually beat Australia in a Test Match!

What advice would you give to anyone who wants to be happy?

Sorry but I couldn't ever answer that question ... I'm now getting serious here ... because there are too many people in this country living in poverty and bringing up kids, sometimes single-handedly, who have so little money they have to use food banks to fill tummies, and wonder every day how they will cope with the next day and can never ever look forward to things like holidays or simple luxuries. What advice could I possibly give them?

Part 2: Work, money and spending

Income

Research study 📁

Title: The Happiness–Income Paradox Revisited

Year: 2010

Country: Various

This study from the US produced new evidence of a phenomenon known to researchers as the happiness–income paradox. At any single point in time, happiness varies directly with income. This is seen both within individual countries and between countries. One would imagine, therefore, that making countries richer would be an effective way to improve the happiness of the people living in them. Research shows, however, that when a nation's income increases, its population doesn't become any happier.

This paradox had been mainly demonstrated using data from developed nations. In this study, researchers sought to establish whether it applied to a wider variety of countries. They used historical data from several international datasets for a total of fifty-four countries, including some from Latin America, Asia, Eastern Europe and Africa, with a mix of economy types. Life satisfaction and financial satisfaction were used as measures of happiness, depending on what data had been collected in the different countries. Data on the annual rate of change in real gross domestic product (GDP) per capita was used to indicate national wealth.

The analysis showed that across the range of countries, the happiness of the population is related to national income in the short term – falling when the economy worsens and improving when it picks up. Over the long term (ten or more years), however, there is no relationship between the two.

Happiness hint ☑

Seek to boost your own income but don't rely on overall improvements in the economy to make you happier in the long term.

Yeah, I'm not sure the economy has much effect on my happiness. But, weirdly, fear of the economy tanking *does* cause me anxiety. Because of all the scaremongering news stories in the UK, I worried that in the event of a no-deal Brexit we would have no fresh fruit and veg and no clean drinking water.

I therefore stockpiled four hundred cans and bottles in the shed. Tomatoes, peaches, beans, bottled water – if it was available to buy and seemed prudent, I stockpiled it.

A year after leaving the EU, although occasional shortages and distribution problems have been reported, everything I stockpiled is still typically available on supermarket shelves, and I still have a very full shed. We did have a day when the water supply was down in East London, though, so the bottled water came in very handy.

But it's fear of energy prices rising and other increases in the cost of living that are scaring me and many other people on low incomes right now. Because no matter what a nation's GDP is per capita, it's still going to benefit the richest more than the poor – we'll most likely stay poor. And not being able to afford to turn the heating on is a deeply miserable state of affairs.

Reference:

Easterlin R.A., McVey L.A., Switek M., Sawangfa O., Zweig J.S., The happiness–income paradox revisited. *Proc Natl Acad Sci USA.* 2010;107(52):22463–8.

Having money in the bank

Research study 🗁

Title: How Your Bank Balance Buys Happiness: The Importance of 'Cash on Hand' to Life Satisfaction

Year: 2016

Country: UK

Having more money in the bank is something that many people would rank highly on the list of things that they think would make them happier. Being wealthy or having a high income and having lots of money in the bank don't necessarily go together, however. Wealth can be tied up in property and investments, and a high income can be matched by equally high outgoings. Researchers from the UK and US undertook this study to find out specifically whether having more liquid wealth, or 'cash on hand', is itself linked with greater happiness.

They collected data in 2014 from customers of a large national bank in the UK who agreed to complete a survey and have the results linked to information about their finances provided by the bank. Around 150,000 bank customers were originally invited to take part. After discounting those who did not have an active account with the bank for the preceding twelve months and those who had their primary account with another bank, the researchers were left with 585 willing and eligible participants, ranging from eighteen to seventy-five years old.

Data was collected on life satisfaction using a set of standard questions as well as participants' perceptions of how comfortable they felt with their finances. Information was also gathered pertaining to income, spending, investments, debt, employment status and relationship status. The participants' liquid wealth was measured by taking a monthly average of how much money they had in their bank accounts on the first day of each month.

The analysis of the data showed that people with higher liquid wealth (more cash in the bank) were generally less worried about their finances, which, in turn, was linked with a greater sense of life satisfaction. This was still the case after taking account of the size of people's spending, investments and debt, as well as other key characteristics which can affect happiness, such as age.

The results showed that it wasn't necessary to have a large amount of cash in the bank in order to experience the benefit. Rather, the effect was greater for people with smaller amounts of liquid wealth. Going from having £1 to £1,000 in the bank led to an average increase of two points on the twenty-point life satisfaction scale. An increase from £1,000 to £10,000, on the other hand, was associated with only a 0.7 point gain in life satisfaction. It wasn't only people with low incomes who experienced a beneficial effect, however. Even high earners with large investments and no debt were happier if some of their wealth was easily accessible.

The researchers concluded that having a minimum buffer of cash in the bank has a notable impact on how satisfied we feel with our lives, resulting from a greater sense of financial security. Above that minimum sufficiency level, the amount of cash in the bank seems to be relatively unimportant in determining happiness.

Happiness hint ☑

If you can, try to keep a minimum buffer of cash in the bank rather than spending your entire income or putting all your spare money into investments where it's not readily accessible.

Oh gosh, having a cash buffer makes all the difference. It's knowing that, if the roof leaks, you can afford to get it fixed rather than have the ceiling drip on your head, and if the boiler breaks you have enough money for a new one rather than having to shiver in four extra layers. It's being able to afford nice Christmas and birthday presents for the kids, and little luxuries if something takes your fancy.

I think it's true what they say: being a billionaire doesn't make you much happier than being comfortable, but being comfortable makes you a lot happier than being in the red. It's having a sense of security, isn't it? The knowledge that, if the worst comes to pass financially and you lose your job or income, you'll still be okay for a bit.

It also means you can take a few risks, rather than having to live sensibly all the time. If you have an idea for a small business, you can put a little capital behind it; if a friend or relative has fallen on hard times, you can afford to help them out.

Also, I think being a billionaire must suck quite a lot. You'd never know whether friends like you for you or your money, and people expect you to solve all the world's problems with the latter. Plus there's a widespread belief that you're evil for the massive disparity between your wealth and the poverty of the starving masses.

So yeah, I'm not sure being filthy rich is all it's cracked up to be, but as the saying goes: I'd like the chance to find out.

Reference:
Ruberton P.M., Lyubomirsky S., Gladstone J., How your bank balance buys happiness: The importance of 'cash on hand' to life satisfaction. *Emotion.* 2016;16(5):575–80.

Being relatively well off

Research study 🗁

Title: Relative Income and Happiness in Asia: Evidence from
Nationwide Surveys in China, Japan, and Korea

Year: 2011

Country: Various

All of us need a certain amount of income to meet our basic material
needs. Typically, though, we judge our level of income not only by
whether it's sufficient but also by how it compares with other people's.

This study explored the relationship between relative income (a
person's income compared to that of others) and how happy people
perceived themselves to be. The researchers wanted to see whether
these two things were similarly related in China, Japan and Korea, as
well as the US.

The study used existing data from broadly comparable nationwide
surveys conducted in each of these countries in 2006. It included
responses from around 1,200 respondents in both Japan and Korea,
around 2,200 in the US and around 2,800 in China – all aged twenty
to sixty-nine. From the surveys, the researchers looked at data on
happiness, individual and family income, which social class people
perceived themselves to be in and where people believed their family

income ranked in their society as a whole (i.e. whether they thought their own family was better or worse off compared with others). In the analysis they also took account of a number of other factors which can influence happiness, including age, sex, number of children, marital status and employment.

The results showed that in all four countries, the size of people's incomes compared to the rest of their society was significantly related to how happy they were. Even when people's perceptions of their social class status were taken into account in the analysis, this relationship still held up. These findings were consistent with earlier studies in Western countries, which also found that relative income is important for happiness.

The study provides evidence to support the theory that our happiness is affected by changes in the gap between our own income and that of others. According to this theory, even if our individual income rises our happiness can be reduced if the income of those we compare ourselves to goes up more.

Happiness hint ☑

Live in a society where most other people have a lower income than you.

Hmm. How am I supposed to arrange that?

I'll just tell my eleven-year-old, 'Come on, Lily, we're moving to Mumbai! That's where your great-grandad was born, though it was called Bombay then, like the potatoes. No, none of your friends will be there but you'll make new ones! Of course your dad won't be okay with it, we'll just abscond and hope he doesn't realise until we're on the flight.'

I mean, I think increasing my income is more viable. It's cool, though, because I'm going to be a pop star soon, so money will be no object.

And even if I don't become a global superstar (let's face it, I can't really tour and break America when I have an eleven-year-old at school), I'll still be happier because I'll be living out my dreams.

Though if this study's correct, I should really just hang out with my old friends and not make friends with pop stars like Bono, because my happiness will suffer when I compare myself to him. It's also best not to get too close to the Edge.

Reference:

Oshio T., Nozaki K., Kobayashi M., Relative Income and Happiness in Asia: Evidence from Nationwide Surveys in China, Japan, and Korea. *Soc Indic Res.* 2011;104(3):351–67.

The Happiness Interview: Kia Abdullah

Kia Abdullah is the bestselling author of three novels: Take It Back, *a* Guardian *and* Telegraph *thriller of the year;* Truth Be Told, *which was shortlisted for a Diverse Book Award; and* Next of Kin, *a* Times *Book of the Month (all published by HarperCollins). She has been awarded a J. B. Priestley Award for Writers of Promise (Royal Literary Fund, 2020) and has written for the* New York Times, *the* Guardian, *the* Financial Times, The Times, *the* Daily Telegraph *and the BBC. She is also the founder of Asian Booklist, a non-profit that advocates for diversity in publishing.*

What three things make you happiest?

Family: I'm happiest when spending time with my partner and my family. As with any close family, we have built a patchwork of in-jokes, catchphrases, shorthand and portmanteaus, which really make me feel a part of something. For example, nearly twenty years ago, I was babysitting my nephews and joked that they were behaving like abysmal kids. 'What are bysmals?' asked one of them. To this day, my family uses 'bysmals' as a collective noun for my nieces and nephews. This sort of shared code gives me a sense of belonging that's vital to my happiness.

Hygge: The Danish concept of 'hygge' became popular a few years ago and is described as 'a quality of cosiness and comfortable conviviality that engenders a feeling of contentment or wellbeing'. We hear a lot about mental health, physical fitness, clean eating, and so on, but nourishing the body on a tactile level is also important. I love wrapping up in soft fabrics and fleecy blankets. We use these materials to soothe babies and young children, but we swap to jeans and stiff, starchy clothes when we're older. Why? I'd live my whole life in fleece if I could.

Nature: I grew up in inner-city London and never fully appreciated the benefits of being in nature. As an adult, I've travelled to some wild and remote places like the Faroe Islands in the North Atlantic, Tanna Island in Vanuatu and the Simien Mountains in Ethiopia. Being in these vast, dramatic landscapes energises me in a way urban living cannot.

What three things would make you happier?

Money: Money is such a clichéd answer and I'm well aware of the research that says happiness plateaus at a certain point but, for me, money facilitates the things that make me happiest. Money means I can buy a house in London to be closer to my family. It means I can buy things for that home that make me physically comfortable. It means I can have a large garden and spend more time outside. It's important, however, to be clear on what you want from your money and to appreciate it when you get it. Otherwise, the goalposts will forever move.

Exercise: If I do thirty minutes of exercise in the morning, I'm much happier and lighter for the rest of the day. The problem is, of course, that I often can't motivate myself to get to the start point. I recently read a tweet that said, 'Is the fucking secret to a happy life just taking a long walk every morning? Is this some kind of joke?' And I laughed because it's true!

Time away from social media: If comparison is the thief of joy, then social media is its funeral pyre. I might be having a perfectly lovely day, but then I'll see something on social media – a harrowing headline, an angry exchange, a sarky remark or even an acquaintance achieving something I haven't managed yet – and it will colour my mood. Time away from social media would definitely make me happier.

What advice would you give to anyone who wants to be happy?

Twain put it well when he said, 'Twenty years from now you will be more disappointed by the things that you didn't do than by the ones you did do.' For me, this is the key to living a happy and fulfilling life.

Career success

Research study 🗀

Title: Does Happiness Promote Career Success? Revisiting the Evidence

Year: 2018

Country: Various

The idea that career success is a prerequisite for lasting happiness is one that many of us had drilled into us as children. Academic research has also supported this idea, with studies showing that happy people tend to earn more money, perform better at work and be rated more favourably by their supervisors.

In 2008, two researchers in the US published a review of the evidence on this topic. They examined the findings of multiple studies and concluded that it was equally plausible that happiness was the cause of career success, rather than the other way around. Ten years later, they repeated this exercise, adding new research which had been undertaken in the intervening period and including a variety of study types with different strengths and weaknesses.

First, they highlighted studies which demonstrated a correlation between happiness and various indicators of success, including job satisfaction, job performance and income. They showed that happy people are less likely to experience burn-out at work and are perceived more positively by their peers and supervisors. Then they looked at studies which measured people's happiness and career status at different points in time. The findings of these studies indicated that happy people are more likely in the future to find employment, feel satisfied with their jobs, perform well and be well regarded in the workplace, and earn more money than unhappy people.

A limitation of both of these study types is that some other unknown factor could still explain the link between happiness and work success. For this reason, the evidence review also included studies in which participants were randomly assigned to two groups, one group was made to feel happier than the other, and then both groups were tested to see how they performed in certain tasks. Results from this type of study showed that people who feel happier have more confidence in their own abilities, which then leads them to perform better. Feeling happy appeared to make people more effective negotiators than less happy people, for example. The researchers speculated that this self-fulfilling prophecy could explain why happy people seem to perform better in the workplace and go further in their careers.

Overall, this review of evidence from multiple research studies mainly concluded that happiness is a cause of career success. It also found evidence, however, that once success is achieved, this causes a further increase in happiness.

Happiness hint ☑

Don't rely on pursuing a promotion to cure your unhappiness. Use other ways to become happy and you may find that both career success and further happiness follow.

I agree with this study, and think just being employed in a job you enjoy can be a cause of happiness. My last proper day job, where I went into the office and wrote entertainment stories for a living, was so much fun that I couldn't wait to get to work in the mornings.

It helped that I really liked my colleagues and was earning £350 a day. The money made me feel valued, and the camaraderie was cheering. This all propelled me to churn out good stories for which I was then praised, so my happiness boosted my career success.

Contrast this with a job I took after this where I only lasted two days, because the atmosphere was toxic, making me so stressed I couldn't concentrate on work. So I concur: it's hard to be successful in a job if you're deeply miserable there.

But it's also true that career success boosts happiness: just ask any author who has just clinched a book deal. Of course, this initial burst of happiness can fade, especially if the books aren't successful, but being able to tell people you're a published author never gets old.

Do you think your happiness has boosted your success at work – or, perhaps, the reverse?

Reference:
Walsh L.C., Boehm J.K., Lyubomirsky S., Does Happiness Promote Career Success? Revisiting the Evidence. *J Career Assess.* 2018;26(2):199–219.

Self-employment

Research study 🗁

Title: How Satisfied are the Self-Employed? A Life Domain View

Year: 2015

Country: Germany

Many of us have considered whether we would be happier working for ourselves rather than an employer. Being your own boss brings freedom from having to meet the demands and expectations of a manager, but potentially also brings different types of responsibility and financial uncertainty. There's plenty of evidence that people who work for themselves tend to have greater job satisfaction, but less research on the question of whether this makes them happier in life generally.

To find out whether self-employed people tend to feel more satisfied overall with their lives, researchers analysed existing data from a large annual survey of Germany's population called the German Socio-Economic Panel. The survey has been running since 1984, collecting data from thousands of households and individuals to track social and economic change in the country.

Some of the questions in the survey have changed over time, so the researchers used data collected between 1997 and 2010 in order to be able to look in a consistent way at all of the different things they were interested in. The data included responses to questions on how satisfied people were with their life and work, their health and employment status. The annual nature of the survey meant that they were able to look at how responses changed over time among people who switched from employment or unemployment into self-employment. They were also able to compare results from people who had become self-employed out of choice and those who had been forced into self-employment through necessity. For the purpose of the study, people were classed as 'self-employed' if they worked full time and defined themselves as self-employed, freelance or working in their family business.

The analysis showed that the reason why people became self-employed mattered when it comes to happiness. Becoming self-employed did lead to greater satisfaction with life overall for those who did so through choice. Those who started working for themselves out of necessity, however, didn't experience the same benefit.

Happiness hint ☑

Consider working for yourself – but only if you really want to.

When I was a kid, my ambitions were all creative. Aged four, we were asked at school to say what we wanted to be when we grew up. I scrawled confidently on a piece of sugar paper that I wanted to be an artist. The teacher wrote, 'What *kind* of artist?' and I replied indignantly, 'A DRAWRING artist!' [sic]. What other kind of artist *was* there?

Then at six, I decided I wanted to write books for a living – and finally, aged twelve, I imagined I'd be a pop star, as I loved writing songs so much. I decided being a pop star was my ultimate dream, and it still is, though I put that dream on hold for years and am only starting to realise it now.

Fast-forward thirty years and I've been self-employed for nearly two decades, and have the grey hair to prove it. I've earned the bulk of my money from writing, though I've also made money from art and design and pop songs. I've always been a creative, and the idea of working in an uncreative role fills me with horror.

Of course, there are things that aren't so great about self-employment. The insecurity, lack of money and having to do your own taxes don't make me orgasm with pleasure, and neither do my regular appointments with the Universal Credit people (to be honest, it would be weird having an orgasm in the Jobcentre, and they'd almost certainly frown upon it, though it might liven up their day).

There's no sick pay, no holiday pay and no guarantee of work. People don't always pay you on time; clients come and go.

But three things make self-employment worthwhile: firstly, you generally get to do what you want for a living. I've been paid for making jokes, writing telly scripts, performing stand-up, singing songs I've written, writing funny books, designing book covers, writing and producing an album of comedy pop songs, scripting and presenting a video series about Twitter for the *Guardian*, travelling the world and writing about it for *The Sunday Times*, and now I've produced the most bomb-ass pop album you've ever heard. The diversity of projects I've worked on and the sheer fun I've had makes me very happy.

Secondly, your time is your own. If you want to take the day off, or the week, or even the month, then you can. You don't need to ask your boss, negotiate time off around other colleagues' holidays, or log it in a spreadsheet as annual leave.

And lastly, while the financial rewards are generally far less than you'd get in a day job for an employer, there's always the possibility of making it really big, especially with a pop career. I dream of living in a beautiful glass house in the Hollywood Hills, waking each day to the glorious California sunshine.

And let's be honest, the average day job ain't gonna get me there.

Reference:

Binder M., Coad A., How Satisfied are the Self-Employed? A Life Domain View. *J Happiness Stud*. 2016;17:1409–33.

Commuting

Research study 📂

Title: Mood During Commute in the Netherlands:
What Way of Travel Feels Best for What Kind of People?

Year: 2017

Country: The Netherlands

Lots of us associate commuting with unhappiness, the mere mention of the word conjuring up images of glum faces on delayed, overcrowded trains and traffic-jam nightmares. Although the COVID-19 pandemic led to a shift to working from home for some, the commute to work remains a fact of everyday life for many.

To understand whether commuting really makes us less happy and whether some methods of commuting affect happiness more than others, researchers analysed existing data on five thousand people in the Netherlands. Participants in the Dutch 'Happiness Indicator' study had recorded what they'd done the previous day and how happy they'd felt at the time in an online diary, making it possible to compare how they felt when at home and how they felt while commuting.

The analysis of the data showed that the participants tended to be less happy during the commute than when they were at home; however, the extent of the difference varied depending on the mode of transport.

Commuting by public transport led to the largest reduction in happiness, while those who commuted by bicycle experienced the smallest reduction. It also turned out that the duration of the commute didn't in itself determine the size of the impact on happiness. Rather, it was the combination of commuting time and the mode of transport that was important. The researchers concluded that some people who commuted by bicycle could even experience an increase in happiness if their commuting time was extended. They also discovered that there was no single universal optimal commuting type – what was best for one person's happiness might not be for another's. Most were happier when commuting with someone else, but some felt better when commuting alone. Similarly, there was a roughly even split between those who should commute outside of rush hour to optimise happiness and those who needed to travel during rush hour to achieve the same effect.

The researchers acknowledged that the participants weren't representative of the general population – most were women and in paid employment, and the majority were highly educated. Therefore, while the study demonstrated that there is no 'one size fits all' approach when it comes to reducing the negative impact of commuting on happiness, it can't tell us which types of commuting are best for different types of people.

Happiness hint ☑

If you can't avoid commuting, test out different modes of transport and shifting the times you travel to find the optimal approach for your wellbeing, if possible. Changing whether you travel alone or in company may also have an effect.

Commuting

Commuting when you're five foot two generally means standing with your face smushed into the armpit of a tall man who smells like a biological weapon.

Speaking of which, I was always so scared of terror attacks that, in my last job, I used to take a twenty-pound taxi into the office in London rather than risk taking the Tube. I knew rationally there was only a tiny chance of getting caught up in a terror attack, but I'm not sure anxiety always responds to logic.

Even taking potential exploding loonies out of the equation, I hated rush-hour commuting. It was physically tiring having to stand for the whole journey (until I piled on the weight, when everyone was keen to give the 'pregnant' woman their seat and I just took it, because there are no other perks to being fat).

There's also an inbuilt awkwardness to so many people being pressed together in such a small space. When your boobs are being pushed by the motion of the train into a random passenger's back, you don't really feel like making eye contact with strangers, let alone talking. So everyone stands there in silence waiting for the ordeal to be over.

I would always just put my headphones on and close my eyes, meaning that I couldn't hear or see any preaching by a religious devotee, or shouting from a crazy person (arguably the same thing). It was just me and the music, though it did mean I occasionally missed my stop.

I can understand why cyclists are happier than people who commute using public transport, but cycling in a city is also quite dangerous. You could wind up splatted on the front of a bus, tomato ketchup on the concrete hamburger of the roads.

And who wants to end up as a condiment?

Reference:
Lancée S., Veenhoven R., Burger M., Mood during commute in the Netherlands: What way of travel feels best for what kind of people? *Transp Res Part A Policy Pract.* 2017;104(2017):195–208.

The Happiness Interview: Jemma Forte

Jemma is a writer and broadcaster. She began her career at the Disney Channel and went on to host shows for ITV, BBC Two and BBC One, including BAFTA-winning children's show Sub Zero, *and the National Lottery with Julian Clary. Jemma currently appears regularly as a contributor on* Jeremy Vine *and* Sky Papers *and also represents luxury soap brand Molton Brown on QVC. She has written five novels and her latest,* Be Careful What You Swipe For *(Neilson, 2020), has resulted in writing frequently for* The Times *on the subject of dating. Jemma lives in London with her two teenage children.*

What three things make you happiest?

Having things in the diary to look forward to.

Earning money from doing things I enjoy and not always working five days a week. Being freelance has its downsides, of course, but being able to do exercise or go shopping at non-peak times is lovely. As is not having to cram all my chores into the weekend. I like that every week is different, too.

People – friends and family. I definitely get my energy from people; I learned that in lockdown, for sure. These days I surround myself with radiators, not drains: people who leave you feeling better when you see them, not worse. I am grateful to be old enough to be able to recognise the difference!

What three things would make you happier?

Boris Johnson and his cronies being voted out. I loathe this government specifically, they are so corrupt and have done so much damage.

Being able to drink wine without putting on weight. This is something which has only kicked in in my forties. It's so dull. I love wine.

Climate change being halted – Brazil not burning down any more of the Amazon rainforest, the equivalent of a 'fishing ceasefire' until the oceans have replenished being mandated. Ideological things which won't happen, but which would stop the constant shadow of a crisis, which can feel very overwhelming. There's so much onus on individuals taking responsibility but the issue is bigger than that. It would be lovely if the world leaders magically turned into superheroes and agreed to do what it takes to ensure a healthy planet and to hell with world economies. Like I said, not going to happen.

Interesting to note that the things which would make me happier are things I have no control over. In a way this pleases me. I think we all have to take responsibility for our own happiness. It's not automatic and no one else can 'make' you happy.

What advice would you give to anyone who wants to be happy?

Being happy isn't a constant state – like everything in life it's something you have to put some effort into. But care less – being embarrassed is a waste of time – and stop worrying about what others are thinking or doing. Notice the small things; be grateful for what you have. When you're stressed or fretting, remember that your thoughts aren't real! If all else fails, switch off the news and have a dance around the kitchen.

Finding happiness outside of work

Research study 📂

Title: Happiness among the Garbage: Differences in Overall
Happiness among Trash Pickers in León (Nicaragua)

Year: 2013

Country: Nicaragua

Given how income and employment can influence wellbeing, it's a
common assumption that those in the most low-status and low-paid
jobs will struggle to achieve happiness. To explore this idea, Spanish
researchers looked at happiness levels among people making their living
in Nicaraguan garbage dumps – a heavily stigmatised group living in
extreme poverty.

They interviewed ninety-nine people whose work consisted of sifting
through garbage to find items that could be sold for recycling, such as
plastic, metal and glass. The workers would also pick out items from
the dump for their own consumption, including food and clothing.

The researchers recorded basic information, such as age, and asked the
participants questions about a range of topics including home life, education, income, social support, leisure time and health, as well as asking
them about their overall happiness and expectations for the future.

Around a quarter of the group were women, with an average age of thirty-seven, while the men had an average age of thirty-two. Three were under the age of sixteen. The vast majority had children (an average of three) and over half had had their first child before they were eighteen. Only 16% of the group had completed primary education and a third were unable to read or write. Over half earned less than forty dollars a month.

The researchers were surprised to find that the vast majority of participants reported being happy and had a positive outlook for the future. The results showed that their access to consumer goods, such as electricity or a mobile phone, and even access to clothing and medicine, were unrelated to whether they were happy. Only having sufficient resources to obtain food proved to be related to happiness, though many said they were happy even when struggling to meet this most basic need.

Happiness was more common among those who reported being in better health, men and those who'd had children at an older age. It also turned out that those who read or played sports in their spare time were more likely to be happy. The researchers concluded that the impact on wellbeing of the stigma, poverty and hardship associated with working at the dump was offset by sources of happiness in other areas of life.

Happiness hint ☑

If your employment and financial circumstances aren't helping, you can still achieve happiness by staying in good health and spending time on rewarding personal relationships and leisure activities.

Well, this study certainly puts my woes into perspective. My career may not yet be setting the world alight, but at least I'm not sifting through rubbish at a tip for less than forty dollars a month. I can see myself struggling to explain that to a snooty partygoer: 'What do you do for a living?' 'I trawl through stinky garbage to find stuff I can flog.' 'Ah, I think I see someone else over there I need to talk to!'

It may not be a high-status job, but I can also imagine that it could be fun, like rooting through bric-a-brac at a jumble sale: you never know when you're going to stumble across a gem someone's discarded. One person's trash is another person's treasure, after all. Plus it's physical exercise, which creates endorphins (which also explains the pleasure created by after-hours sports playing). And at least there's no boss looking over your shoulder, ready to berate you for slacking.

Being in good health is, of course, a major contributor to happiness. It's hard to feel happy when you're in pain, full of cold or nauseous. Kieran has several long-term chronic illnesses including asthma, fibromyalgia, IBS and arthritis, and though he manages them well by listening to his body, they place physical limitations on him – though, unusually, they don't seem to affect his happiness. He's a very happy person, though who knows – maybe he'd be the happiest person in the world if he were in better health?

As for pursuits in your spare time making you happy: it's a lovely revelation that even in the lowliest job, you can find happiness from your non-work pursuits. And I'm not surprised that reading cheered participants up. Especially if they were reading my books!

What hobbies make you happy? What would you do in your spare time if time, money, space and resources were no object?

Reference:

Vázquez J.J., Happiness among the garbage: Differences in overall happiness among trash pickers in León (Nicaragua). *J Posit Psychol.* 2013;8(1):1–11. doi:10.1080/17439760.2012.743574

Consumption

Research study 🗁

Title: Does Consumption Buy Happiness? Evidence from the
        United States

Year: 2010

Country: USA

We all know that buying things can give us a rush of excitement but whether it leads to more than momentary happiness is the critical question.

There are reasons to speculate that the consumption of goods may increase our sense of wellbeing – it may result in us acquiring things which reduce material hardship and make our lives easier, or it may give us status symbols which make us feel better about our place in society and reduce a sense of inferiority to others. Another notion, which the researchers in this study chose to explore, is that consumption may improve happiness because of an effect it has on our social relationships.

They used existing data from the long-running US Health and Retirement Study, which provides a nationally representative picture of the country's population over the age of fifty. The researchers' objective was to examine the relationship between happiness and various types of consumption expenditure. The analysis included data from 1,733 respondents who had answered questions on their consumption, happiness and other psychological factors in 2006. Annual consumption expenditure was split into nine categories:

- Leisure (e.g. hobbies, holidays, sport and exercise, and tickets to shows, movies and events)

- Durables (e.g. domestic appliances, TVs and computers)

- Charity and gifts to family and friends outside the household

- Personal care and clothing (e.g. housekeeping supplies, dry cleaning, gardening, clothing and hairdressing)

- Health care (e.g. medications and health insurance)

- Food and drink consumed at home

- Eating (and drinking) out

- Utilities and housing (e.g. mortgage/rent, household bills, furnishings and home repairs)

- Vehicles

The researchers found that only one type of consumption was positively related to happiness – leisure consumption. The people who spent more on leisure tended to be happier. The analysis also showed that that connection between leisure consumption and happiness was partially accounted for by its positive effect on social connectedness. Those who spent more money on leisure consumption generally spent more time engaged in social activities and felt less lonely.

The study provides some evidence to suggest that spending more on leisure activities might lead to greater happiness, but it doesn't prove this. It could be that when people are happier they feel more like participating in leisure activities. It's also important to acknowledge that the participants of the study were older than the general population, with an average age of sixty-six. At different stages of life, other types of consumption may be associated with happiness.

Happiness hint ☑

Spend your disposable income on leisure activities, rather than flashy cars, expensive clothing or a fancy new fridge.

I've read this a lot: that buying *experiences* is a better use of your money than buying *things*. I actually have very little disposable cash at present – and what scant money I have, I need to save for home emergencies, finishing my debut pop album and my daughter Lily's birthday presents – so it's not a choice I'm making right now.

However, Lily's eleventh birthday is coming up, and for once I'm departing from purchasing the usual flurry of presents in favour of buying her two experiences: 'Meet the Monkeys' at London Zoo, and getting her ears pierced for the first time.

Meeting and being able to hold and feed cute little monkeys will be priceless. The experience will only last twenty minutes, but my own little monkey will be able to relive it through her memories of it, telling people about it and when she looks back at the photos and videos of the event.

Getting her ears pierced might not be as enjoyable at the time, but it's a rite of passage which will enable Lil to raid my extensive costume jewellery collection, so I'm sure it'll be worth the few seconds of pain.

I think these experiences will be worth the £250 they're going to cost, even though Lil's fifty-five years off being sixty-six. It's worth mentioning that, while spending money on health care might bring no happiness, being healthy does make you happy, which is a bit of a contradiction.

Likewise, spending on vehicles might not bring you joy, but taking the car instead of commuting on public transport might. And eating out isn't a fun thing to pay for, but the experience of having dinner with your loved ones is.

But back to leisure: what kind of leisure experiences would you like to try?

Reference:
DeLeire T., Kalil A., Does consumption buy happiness?
Evidence from the United States. *Int Rev Econ*. 2010;57(2):163–76.

Shopping online

Research study 📁

Title: Click It and Buy Happiness: Does Online Shopping Improve Subjective Well-being of Rural Residents in China?

Year: 2021

Country: China

Online shopping makes our lives a lot easier by allowing us to easily buy the things we need without leaving the house. As well as saving us time by doing away with the need to physically go to shops looking for the things we want, it also enables us to discover products we wouldn't have otherwise known about and to easily buy things which aren't available locally. Focused specifically on rural China, this study investigated whether the benefits of online shopping made people happier.

They used data collected by a survey in 2019, along with some face-to-face interviews. In total, they collected data from 813 people, including information on basic characteristics such as age, gender and income, as well as living conditions, online shopping habits and expenditure. Respondents were also asked to rate their own happiness and level of satisfaction with their lives.

In analysing the data, the researchers used an approach designed to take account of the fact that online shoppers were typically different from non-online shoppers in other ways which might influence their level of happiness; for example, they tended to be younger, better educated and were more likely to own a car.

Of the 813 respondents, 321 stated that they shopped online. The results showed that online shopping was associated with greater happiness and satisfaction with life. The more people spent shopping online, the happier they were and those with the lowest household incomes benefitted the most.

The respondents used online shopping to buy a variety of types of goods; however, the researchers didn't look into whether the benefits differed depending on what was purchased. We also don't know if these findings reflect specific circumstances which apply to the rural population of China or whether the same apparent benefits of online shopping apply to people living in other parts of the world.

Happiness hint ☑

If you live in a rural area, try shopping online more.

I do love online shopping. I can't really afford anything at present, so I've created an online wish list. Any time I want to buy something, I simply add the item to the list instead of purchasing it, and when it comes to my birthday or Christmas, my lovely patrons buy me the gifts. It's so nice to know that there are people who care about me enough to buy me stuff I want or need. It might be worth creating a wish list for your own friends and family if you're skint, as you'll probably get generic gifts you don't especially want (like bath sets and candles) if you don't!

I don't live in rural China – far from it – but online shopping provides a dopamine rush which I'm sure applies to thousands of different cultures. I'm perplexed by this line, though: 'The more people spent shopping

116

online, the happier they were and those with the lowest household incomes benefitted the most.' Surely the more you spend on a low income, the less money you have and the more stressed out you feel?!

I highly recommend that these people create a wish list instead.

During the Covid lockdowns, many people were forced to increase the amount they shopped online, or started shopping online for the first time, due to retail store closures and fear of social contact.' Although they probably weren't all happy about that, retail industry research published in 2020 showed that 44% of UK shoppers were anticipating a permanent shift in the way they shopped and 47% were expecting to shop online more frequently, so it must have been doing something for them.''

Reference:

Zheng H., Ma W., Click it and buy happiness: does online shopping improve subjective well-being of rural residents in China? *Appl Econ.* 2021. doi:10.1080/00036846.2021.1897513

---

*   https://blog.ons.gov.uk/2020/09/18/how-the-covid-19-pandemic-has-accelerated-the-shift-to-online-spending/

**   https://www.retailgazette.co.uk/blog/2020/08/almost-half-consumers-permanently-change-shopping-habits-post-covid/

The Happiness Interview: Alom Shaha

Alom Shaha is the author of books including The Young Atheist's Handbook *and* Mr Shaha's Recipes for Wonder *(Scribble UK, 2018). As well as writing books, he has created, written, produced, directed and appeared in a wide range of science communication projects, ranging from TV series to live science shows. He is a dad of two and teaches part-time at a comprehensive school.*

What three things make you happiest?

Being a parent, spending time with my children and watching them being happy and enjoying themselves.

Seeing other people I love being happy.

Accomplishing 'creative' stuff.

What three things would make you happier?

The certain knowledge that I am going to live long enough to see my children grow old and have happy and contented lives.

Feeling better rested, and more healthy.

Completing more 'creative' stuff.

What advice would you give to anyone who wants to be happy?

Try to live long enough so that some of the angst and stuff that comes with being young fades away and you discover that 'happiness' really is just about finding a sense of contentedness with who you are.

Consuming luxury goods

Research study 🗁

Title: The Silver Lining of Materialism: The Impact of Luxury
Consumption on Subjective Well-being

Year: 2011

Country: Belgium

Materialistic goals are often linked to people's ideals of perfect happiness. Evidence suggests, though, that those who pursue materialistic goals are unhappier and less satisfied with their lives than people who are less materialistic. The researchers who conducted this study wanted to understand why so many of us still subscribe to materialistic ambitions given that this seems to be linked with unhappiness. They wanted to test out the theory that those who are more materialistic consume more luxury goods and that the consumption of luxury goods creates a boost in happiness which rewards and reinforces this approach to life.

In 2009, they conducted a survey of over two thousand people in the Flemish part of Belgium, ranging in age from sixteen to eighty-eight with a roughly equal split of males and females. The survey collected basic information about the respondents and included questions designed to measure their life satisfaction, tendency to choose luxury brands and materialism. To assess materialism, respondents were asked how much they agreed with various statements, such as: 'The things I own say a lot about how well I'm doing in life.'

The results showed that people who were materialistic tended to consume more luxury goods than those who weren't, and that this consumption of luxury goods led to people feeling happier and more satisfied with their lives as a short-term consequence. It also turned out that this effect was greater for materialistic people. These findings applied irrespective of the respondents' age, sex or income.

The researchers concluded that while materialism itself is not beneficial for mental wellbeing, the consumption of luxury goods that results from it does provide a short-term happiness boost which rewards and reinforces a materialistic outlook.

Happiness hint ☑

Buying luxury goods can give you a quick-fix happiness boost, but you might want to rethink your outlook on life for the longer term if you're generally a materialistic person (the chapters on 'Bought experiences', 'Going on holiday' and 'Acts of kindness' might give you some inspiration).

This is what I wondered about the previous study: how short term is the resulting happiness boost from online shopping? As with this study, I doubt it lasts long.

Also, having read the above: how fragile must your ego be that it needs to be propped up by a Louis Vuitton suitcase?

I like nice things as much as the next person, but it doesn't really matter to me if those things are embossed with Hugo Boss or not. I get that luxury goods might be well made, but so are many non-branded products.

And how well you're doing in life isn't necessarily linked to your salary. I'd have more money if I were stacking the shelves at Asda, so I'd be able to afford luxury goods, but I'd also be as miserable as a goth in a heatwave.

I once spoke to a woman who hated her job as a stockbroker, and asked her why she didn't quit. She gestured to her Prada purse and said, 'I simply couldn't give up this lifestyle.'

Ironically, her lifestyle meant she lived a life she didn't enjoy much, all for the sake of purchasing designer items so that other people could think she was successful. Hating your job isn't my definition of success, even if it allows you to keep up appearances.

Of course, I reserve the right to retract all this when I become a pop star and dress head to toe in Gucci.

Reference:
Hudders L., Pandelaere M., The Silver Lining of Materialism: The Impact of Luxury Consumption on Subjective Well-Being. *J Happiness Stud.* 2012;13(3):411–37.

Decluttering

Research study 📂

Title: In Pursuit of Happiness: Phenomenological Study of the KonMari Decluttering Method

Year: 2017

Country: Unspecified

The idea of decluttering your home to improve your sense of wellbeing gained huge popularity when Japanese organising expert Marie Kondo shot to fame with the publication of her book, *The Life Changing Magic of Tidying Up*, in 2014. While many authors have written self-help books on the subject of decluttering, her 'KonMari' method was notable for explicitly linking the process of deciding what to keep and what to throw away with the question of whether each object elicits a feeling of happiness.

A UK researcher seeking to better understand the relationship between happiness and the ownership and discarding of physical objects interviewed eleven women who had applied the KonMari method in their own lives. Aged from twenty-six to forty-seven, they had each spent between two months and five years trying the approach and had documented their attempts at decluttering through pictures, blogs, diaries or videos. The researcher used these materials to prompt recollections from the participants about their experiences and then analysed their content along with the interview transcripts.

Six of the eleven women reported that they were pure KonMari converts who followed all of its steps faithfully. The rest of the participants said that they had given up at various stages or had deviated from the set method to suit their own preferences. Although they reported having difficulty in keeping on top of the new system for ordering their possessions after the initial declutter, all said that applying KonMari had transformed tidying up from a mundane chore into an experience that triggered happiness.

The researcher found that KonMari's unique approach of symbolically classifying objects according to whether they 'spark joy' disrupts or revitalises our existing relationship with those objects. This experience, she concluded, can induce high levels of happiness and improve wellbeing. It's not clear how much we can generalise from these findings, however, as the study looked at a small number of people and didn't include men.

Happiness hint ☑

Try Marie Kondo's decluttering technique and see if it 'sparks joy'.

What perplexes me is Kondo's expectations of our relationship with everyday household items. Can a bottle of bleach really spark joy? What about a soggy washing-up sponge or a toilet brush? Surely these things are just practical and functional – they're not *supposed* to spark joy, any more than scrubbing the shit-streaked bog is likely to make you feel ecstatic.

I get that clothes, furniture and decorative accessories can spark joy (or not, as the case may be) but dishcloths and kitchen roll just don't elicit that depth of emotion for most people.

So I prefer to use TV presenter Anthea Turner's decluttering mantra: 'Is this beautiful, useful or seriously sentimental? If not, get rid of it.'

That way, all the functional stuff above comes under 'useful', as does anything utilitarian. My daughter's scrawly paintings from when she was a toddler can be filed under 'seriously sentimental', and my costume jewellery under 'beautiful'.

I understand that nobody's done a study on Anthea Turner's words of wisdom yet – but maybe they should?

Reference:
Hsin-Hsuan Meg Lee. In Pursuit of Happiness: Phenomenological Study of the KonMari Decluttering Method. *Adv Consum Res*. 2017;45:454–7.

Bought experiences

Research study 🗁

Title: Happiness for Sale: Do Experiential Purchases Make Consumers Happier than Material Purchases?

Year: 2009

Country: USA

It's been suggested that spending money on experiences rather than material things leads to greater happiness. The idea is that holidays, days out and theatre trips, for example, are ultimately better for our mental wellbeing than indulging in flashy cars or the latest gadgets. To test this out, scientists in the US conducted three experiments. As well as looking at how these two different types of consumption affected happiness they also explored whether it matters how positive or negative the experience is. In addition, they sought to test out a potential mechanism by which experiences might create greater happiness than material purchases.

For the first experiment they recruited 211 students from the University of Texas at Austin who were given extra credit in exchange for taking part. They asked each student to recall a past purchase and how happy they were with it afterwards on a seven-point scale. Some of the students were asked to recall a purchase that they had enjoyed, while others were asked to recall a purchase they had not enjoyed.

The participants were asked how much they spent on the purchase and how long ago they made it – both of which were factored into the analysis. The results from twenty-one of the students had to be discounted because they answered the wrong question – describing enjoyable purchases when asked for unenjoyable ones and vice versa. The analysis of the remaining results showed no notable distinction between the material purchases and experiences in terms of their impact on happiness.

In the second experiment, 198 students were randomly split into two groups. One group were asked to recall and describe three past purchases that had turned out well and the other were asked to recall three past purchases that had turned out poorly. They rated each purchase on a seven-point scale from 'completely material' to 'completely experiential' and answered questions on how happy those purchases made them feel.

The results showed that the level of happiness induced by positive purchases was greater for experiences than material things. The more experiential the purchase, the happier it made them feel. If the purchase was a negative one, however, it didn't make a difference what the nature of it was in terms of its impact on happiness.

The final experiment was designed to test whether this link between how experiential a purchase is and how happy it can make you feel could be explained by how we adapt to experiences compared to material objects. This time 355 students were recruited and split into two groups. One group were told they each had three 'lab dollars' with which they could purchase one experience from a set of three options: a video to watch, a song to listen to or a video game to play. Happiness data was collected from the participants one day, one week and two weeks after the experience in a questionnaire sent by email.

The other group were told they could spend their three lab dollars on one of seven physical items, including a keychain, a deck of cards and a screwdriver. After 'purchasing' an item they were allowed to take it home with them. They completed follow-up questionnaires by email in the same way as the 'experience' group.

The analysis showed that levels of happiness diverged over time depending on whether an experience or material object had been 'purchased'. The scientists concluded that purchasing an experience appeared to have a longer-term impact on happiness than purchasing an object. This meant that while a positive purchase of an experience had a bigger impact on happiness than a positive purchase of an object, a purchase of an experience which was perceived to be negative by the consumer would cause greater unhappiness than a negatively perceived purchase of an object. They argued that it is too simplistic therefore to advise people to consume experiences over material things to achieve greater happiness as a blanket rule – experiences only offer an advantage if they're perceived positively by the consumer. An experience that leaves you feeling negative about it is worse for your happiness than purchasing an object that leaves you feeling negative.

A limitation of this study is that it doesn't show the impact of cumulative purchases over time, although the scientists theorised that a lifetime of negative experiences may be the worst way to spend your money for avoiding unhappiness.

Happiness hint ☑

Spend your money on good experiences rather than objects (but make sure they do turn out to be good ones).

I never used to be a very experience-happy person. Back when I did a lot of online dating, whenever a bloke I was chatting to would suggest an activity date, I would groan inwardly.

I didn't *want* to go to an origami festival, climb a vertiginous wall full of colourful handholds, or be deafened at a rock gig where I was too short to see anything. I just wanted to sit quietly in a café or restaurant, drink green tea and learn about the guy. You can't gaze into each other's eyes when you're staring at a climbing wall.

It seems that I may have been mistaken to take this view, especially when I consider that, whenever I take part in an experience, I usually end up feeling better and cheerier. It also bonds you to the other person as you're sharing the experience.

You can't always predict which experiences are going to be positive. As an anxious, sensitive and physically unfit person, I'd definitely rule out the following: extreme sports, potential danger, death metal concerts, intense physical activity, venomous animals and anything in very cold or wet weather.

But quiet arts and crafts-type stuff is perfect. I wish I'd gone to that origami festival.

Reference:
Nicolao L., Irwin J.R., Goodman J.K., Happiness for Sale:
Do Experiential Purchases Make Consumers Happier than Material
Purchases? *J Consum Res*. 2009;36(2):188–98.

The Happiness Interview: Robin Ince

Robin Ince is a comedian, author, broadcaster and populariser of scientific ideas. The Guardian *once declared him a 'becardiganed polymath', which seems about right. He is probably best known as the co-host of the Sony Gold Award-winning BBC Radio 4 series* The Infinite Monkey Cage *with Professor Brian Cox. He also co-hosts the podcast Book Shambles, with Josie Long, which has over 100,000 listeners a month and is part of The Cosmic Shambles Network, which he also co-created. His book,* I'm a Joke and So Are You, *was described by Chortle as 'one of the best books ever written about what it means to be a comedian'. His latest book is* The Importance of Being Interested: Adventures in Scientific Curiosity *(Atlantic, 2021).*

What three things make you happiest?

Watching my son build sand cars on a summer's day on a quiet beach.

Sitting in a quiet tearoom with a slice of Victoria sponge browsing the contents of a bag of books I have just bought from a second-hand bookshop.

Watching a black-and-white movie in the afternoon with my wife (rare to find such time).

What three things would make you happier?

If I could turn off my inner voice that babbles persistently and anxiously about my past and future failures.

Taking compliments as seriously as I take criticism.

More hot baths.

What advice would you give to anyone who wants to be happy?

To try not to measure yourself against other people, but think about what you want to achieve.

Going on holiday

Research study 🗁

Title: The Effect of Leisure Activities on Life Satisfaction:
The Importance of Holiday Trips

Year: 2011

Country: Germany

Going on holiday is something many of us regard as an effective short-term cure for low mood. The scientific validity of this idea was explored in this study by Dutch researchers using existing data from a large-scale study over time of the German population.

The German Socio-Economic Panel Study began in 1984 and involves asking a sample of the population questions on a range of topics. Participants are interviewed once a year, with questions covering health, education, work and wellbeing, among other things. Questions on leisure activities have not been included every year, so the researchers were only able to use data from 1990, 1995, 1998 and 2003 for their analysis. The number of participants varies each year, with around 20,400 included in 2003.

In the analysis, they looked at the relationships between answers to a question on how satisfied people felt with their lives as a whole and answers to questions on a range of leisure activities, including going on day trips and holidays, as well as things such as playing board games, eating out, attending concerts and visiting neighbours. They also factored in responses to other questions which might account for any relationship between leisure activities and happiness, including personality type, marriage, income, age and health.

The results showed that people who took a holiday trip every year were happier in that year than those who didn't. This applied regardless of personality type, age, sex, health, employment and marital status. The researchers noted that this raised level of happiness was comparable to, or greater than, that achieved by some mood-enhancing interventions or financial windfalls. They suggested that taking a few holiday trips a year could even be more effective than winning £50,000. Any boost in happiness appeared to be short-lived, however. It wasn't possible to determine from the available data exactly how long the effect lasted but they could say that it wasn't more than a year.

Partly contradicting the findings of some other studies, they found no correlation between happiness and any of the other leisure activities they looked at. They noted, however, that this result may have been affected by limitations in the way some of the questions were phrased.

Happiness hint ☑

Go on a few nice day trips and holidays every year.

I can't afford a holiday. My last proper holiday was two weeks in America back in 2017, where I got hitched to the wrong guy and had a fraught honeymoon where we were both miserable. Still, nobody got shot, that's the main thing.

It feels a bit wrong to take holidays when you're self-employed. Not only is any holiday unpaid, eating into your productivity and chances of success, every day is essentially a holiday. My job is fun: I make my own hours and write absolute gibberish for money. If I feel ill, I don't have to phone in sick, because that would mean talking to myself. I just give myself the day off and wait until I feel better to start working again.

Sure, if I were earning £80,000, I'd fly first class to Jamaica with Kieran (his dad's half-Jamaican but Kieran's never been). I'd spend two weeks making love to him in a luxury spa hotel, have deep-tissue massages, eat delicious food and sunbathe under a canopy of palm trees. I'd relish not having to do the washing-up or make the bed.

But I earn closer to £8,000, so my next holiday will be a weekend away with him in Bournemouth. Hey, it's better than nothing.

Reference:
Nawijn J., Veenhoven R., The Effect of Leisure Activities on Life Satisfaction: The Importance of Holiday Trips. In: Brdar I. (ed.), *The Human Pursuit of Well-Being.* Dordrecht: Springer; 2011:39–53.

Winning the lottery

Research study 🗀

Title: Money and Mental Wellbeing: A Longitudinal Study of Medium-sized Lottery Wins

Year: 2006

Country: UK

The question of whether money brings happiness is a constant subject of debate. To explore this scientifically, researchers analysed data from a random sample of British lottery winners. The data was collected through the British Household Panel Survey, in which a nationally representative sample of over five thousand households have been interviewed annually since 1991. All those in the household aged sixteen and over are included.

The survey includes a standard measure of mental wellbeing and also records wins on the lottery or football pools. As lottery wins are far more common than pools wins due to the popularity of the lottery, the researchers referred to all wins as 'lottery wins' for simplicity. The analysis included data on mental wellbeing scores and lottery wins between 1996 and 2003, with adjustment for inflation. The researchers looked at changes in wellbeing from two years prior to a lottery win to two years after.

Focusing on what they termed 'medium-sized wins', they identified a total of 137 winners. These wins ranged in size from £1,000 to around £120,000 in 1998 pounds sterling. When compared both to those who had no wins and those who had smaller wins, this group went on to have significantly better mental wellbeing. Two years after winning, they had experienced an improvement of 1.4 points on a thirty-six-point wellbeing scale.

The study doesn't tell us about the impact of large lottery wins but does provide evidence that a medium-sized lottery win is beneficial for happiness.

Happiness hint ☑

Win a decent amount of money on the lottery.

Ha ha, 'win a decent amount of money on the lottery', like it's within our control! I often fantasise about winning the EuroMillions, which is ridiculous as I don't *play* the EuroMillions. My dad always used to say the lottery was a 'tax on the stupid', and given the odds, I'd tend to agree.

The closest I've ever come to winning the lottery was when my ex convinced me to buy Premium Bonds. One day, I was on the phone to my mate Kia (a bestselling author whose happiness interview is in this very book). We were talking about the improvements she was making to her home, when I received a text saying, 'You are a Premium Bonds winner'.

'Oh my God, Ariane!' Kia squealed. 'You know the top prize is a million pounds?'

'If I've won a million pounds I'll help you with your home improvements,' I promised.

I got off the phone so I could find out how much I'd won. I felt quite deflated to learn it was only twenty-five pounds.

'I won't be able to help you with your home improvements,' I told Kia later.

'Maybe you could buy me a packet of crisps instead?' she suggested.

I agreed, and she asked for sweet-chilli-flavoured crisps, like a good Asian.

I would have bought her the crisps even if I hadn't won the twenty-five pounds.

Reference:
Gardner J., Oswald A.J., Money and Mental Wellbeing: A Longitudinal Study of Medium-sized Lottery Wins. *J Health Econ.* 2007;26(1):49–60.

The Happiness Interview: Mitch Benn

Mitch Benn is a comedian, actor, musician and the author of the acclaimed SF trilogy Terra, Terra's World *and* Terra's War *(Raging Vega Press, 2021). He is probably best known for his long stint as the resident satirical songwriter on BBC Radio 4's* The Now Show. *Mitch contributes a weekly column to the* New European *newspaper. He lives in South West London, has two teenaged kids and far too many guitars.*

What three things make you happiest?

Family, in all its myriad variant forms.

Cats. There's a reason they own the internet.

Making a difficult decision, and then discovering it was the right one.

What three things would make you happier?

I'd like to be able to detoxify my relationship with food.

I'd like to have more confidence in my own decision-making processes.

I'd like the Conservative Party to cease to exist.

What advice would you give to anyone who wants to be happy?

Don't sweat the small stuff. And you may not realise it now, but about 90% of it is small stuff. It's statistically almost inevitable that one day, something will happen to you that will put everything, in the immortal words of Spinal Tap, into 'too much fucking perspective', and whatever pain and grief this event causes you will only be exacerbated by the sudden realisation that you've spent most of your life fretting about stuff that really doesn't matter at all. So why not do yourself a favour and not wait for this bad thing to happen before having this realisation?

Part 3: Health and beauty

Good health

Research study 🗀

Title: The Effects of Chronic Illness on Aspirations and
      Subjective Wellbeing

Year: 2017

Country: Indonesia

Government health campaigns, advertising and the media serve up a
constant stream of information and advice on adopting a healthy lifestyle to reduce the risks of developing long-term illnesses, such as heart
disease, cancer and diabetes. Less talked about is the relationship
between maintaining good physical health and good mental health.
Building on research showing that long-term health conditions and
happiness are closely linked, this study investigated one potential
mechanism which might account for the connection.

Few of us enjoy being ill, but chronic illnesses, such as cancer, can have
a substantial negative impact on other aspects of people's lives, aside
from the obvious effect on their physical health. When people become
too ill to work they may find themselves facing unexpected financial
hardship, especially if they are faced with paying for substantial
medical or care costs. This can add to any restrictions their poor health
has already placed on their social lives and recreation, and create

further stress. A sense of frustration at missing out on aspects of life they would otherwise expect to enjoy may begin to develop.

In this study, the researcher wanted to find out how the impact of having a long-term illness affected people's ability to achieve their personal aspirations and whether this might, in turn, reduce happiness. The data used had been collected in 2007 and 2014 through a national survey in Indonesia covering around 83% of the country's population. The Indonesian Family Life Survey covered more than ten thousand households, with questions on a broad range of subjects, including happiness and living standards. All members of the household aged fifteen and over were included in the survey.

Participants were asked if they had been diagnosed with any of a list of long-term conditions, including, for example, high blood pressure, diabetes, tuberculosis, asthma, cancer, arthritis and heart disease. Those who had were asked when they'd been diagnosed and whether the condition limited their physical activities. Around 5% of adults had a chronic condition that affected their ability to work. The average length of time they'd been suffering from the condition was five and a half years.

The survey also included a question in which respondents were asked where they felt they stood on a six-step imaginary ladder in which the poorest group were at the bottom. They were also asked which step they felt they were on five years ago and which step they expected to be on in five years' time. The data from this question was used to measure the gap between participants' aspirations and their reality.

The analysis of the data showed that being diagnosed with a chronic condition was linked with both a decrease in happiness and an increase in the gap between aspirations and reality. This was due to people lowering their evaluation of their current situation when they became ill, rather than lowering their expectations for the future. As expected, there was also evidence of an impact on future happiness following a diagnosis of a chronic condition. Generally, every one-year increase in the length of time since people had been diagnosed was associated with a subsequent reduction in their level of happiness.

The author of the study concluded that the findings supported the theory that the link between chronic conditions and lower happiness is explained by the increasing gap between people's aspirations and their reality over the duration of the illness.

Happiness hint ☑

Adopt a healthy lifestyle to minimise your chances of developing a long-term health condition. This includes not smoking, limiting your alcohol consumption and following government guidelines on exercise and eating well.

This is unsurprising. I'm lucky in that I only have one debilitating health condition: hypersomnia. I sleep, on average, eleven to twelve hours a day. I inherited it from my dad, who used to sleep so much I would call him 'Our father, who art in bed'.

It only affects my ambitions by decreasing the amount of time I have to spend on them. As a result, I don't watch telly, listen to podcasts or have hobbies. I just work, exercise, sleep and look after Lily.

I'd rather not have hypersomnia but am relieved it's only sleeping to excess and there's no pain or discomfort.

As I've mentioned already, my poor boyfriend Kieran has asthma, fibromyalgia, arthritis, migraines and numerous allergies to things like lactose, pork products and pet hair. He is infirm, though thankfully not *unfirm*.

Weirdly, though, he's one of the happiest, most fulfilled people I know. He's a Buddhist, which might have something to do with it – he's just extremely chilled and philosophical about his illnesses. And he's learned how to manage them by pacing himself and not overdoing it. He knows what he can't change, and focuses on doing things that make him happy in his spare time, even if he only has the energy to do a little every so often. He genuinely seems cheerier than people who are in perfect health, probably because he prioritises doing things that matter to him.

His fibromyalgia also means he has an excuse to ask me for regular massages, so it's not all bad.

Reference:
Lim S.S., The Effects of Chronic Illness on Aspirations and Subjective Wellbeing. *J Happiness Stud*. 2020;21(5):1771–93.

Physical activity

Research study 🗁

Title: Happier People Live More Active Lives: Using Smartphones to Link Happiness and Physical Activity

Year: 2017

Country: Unspecified

The importance of keeping active for physical health is well established. As well as reducing the risk of diseases, such as coronary heart disease and diabetes, exercise can improve mood and reduce the risk of depression. Even normal everyday physical activity we might not think of as exercise, such as using stairs, gardening and walking to the shops, can achieve health benefits. In this study, researchers in the UK sought to find out whether this kind of activity can also improve happiness.

As this kind of everyday physical activity is often brief and something we tend not to give much thought to, just asking people to consciously record or recall how much they've done isn't a very reliable way of measuring it. To get a more accurate picture, the researchers used a smartphone app designed to gather data on people's levels of physical activity and happiness. For users, the benefit of the app was the regular feedback it provided into the context of their own everyday mood changes.

The app was made freely available on the Google Play store in February 2013 and had been used by 12,838 people by the time researchers began analysing the data in June 2014. Most people had provided details of their sex, age and ethnicity. This data showed that slightly more than half of the users were male, the most common age group was twenty-five to thirty-four years old and around two-thirds were white.

The app collected data in a variety of ways. It would send notifications at two random moments in the day explicitly requesting users to answer short questions on their mood and what they were currently doing. Users could also choose to initiate a survey on the app themselves which went into more detail. Each time users unlocked a new stage of the app, they answered questions designed to measure how satisfied they were with their lives. Physical activity was recorded via the phone's accelerometer, as well as users' responses to questions.

The analysis of the data showed a link between physical inactivity and lower happiness. Those who moved more frequently throughout the day, even if that movement wouldn't be classed as rigorous exercise, were generally happier. Ordinary everyday movement, such as walking and fidgeting, was related to feeling better. People also tended to be happier in the specific moments when they were being active. The researchers acknowledged that this study wasn't designed in such a way that it could prove whether greater happiness is really caused by greater levels of activity, rather than the other way around. Despite this limitation, it adds to a body of research suggesting that keeping active could be beneficial for your mental, as well as physical, health.

Happiness hint ☑

Get up and move around more.

Physical activity

It's very frustrating to me that exercise is linked to longevity and happiness, as I'm definitely not happy *while* I'm doing it. I mean, I'm happy *that* I'm doing it because I know it's good for me physically and mentally, and after I've done it I'm like, 'Boom! What a success of a human I am.'

But during it I'm properly clock-watching, counting down the minutes until I can stop. That doesn't really suggest it's an enjoyable activity. I don't make love and check my watch halfway through (though I suppose that is a form of exercise. I'm lazy, though, so usually do it missionary!).

The worst thing about exercise, other than hating the arduous sensations while I'm doing it, is feeling like a failure when I don't do it. If I end the day and have spent it lying in bed like a fat slug, my brain says, 'Congratulations, you have failed at life! You are now destined for a life of chronic disease and self-loathing. Well done.'

And, given the studies, I can't even argue back. I also know alien creatures who love running and cycling, who really get off on the endorphins they produce and feel depressed if they don't have the chance to get out in the fresh air and exercise.

I don't understand them, but they exist.

Reference:
Lathia N., Sandstrom G.M., Mascolo C., Rentfrow P.J., Happier People Live More Active Lives: Using Smartphones to Link Happiness and Physical Activity. *PloS One*. 2017;12(1): e0160589. doi:10.1371/journal.pone.0160589

Avoiding fast food

Research study 📁

Title: Too Impatient to Smell the Roses: Exposure to
    Fast Food Impedes Happiness

Year: 2013

Country: USA

A series of three studies was conducted to test whether the fast food industry has an impact on our ability to experience happiness.

In the first study, 280 native English speakers completed an online survey to measure their tendency to savour emotional responses to enjoyable experiences. The results showed that those who lived in neighbourhoods with a higher concentration of fast food restaurants were less likely to savour everyday pleasurable experiences. This remained the case after taking account of people's age and other neighbourhood characteristics which might explain the link.

In the second study, 257 participants were shown a picture of a burger and fries with a cup of coffee, either in McDonald's packaging or in ceramic tableware. Each group were then asked to rate their happiness on a seven-point scale – some immediately after seeing the food and the rest after first being shown ten photographs of scenic natural beauty. Although simply seeing the food in the McDonald's packaging didn't directly affect happiness, the results indicated that it did reduce the extent to which people savoured and gained happiness from looking at the pleasant scenery.

For the final study, 122 participants were put through a similar experiment in which the photographs were replaced with a beautiful aria. The results were similar, with those who'd been exposed to the classic fast food imagery experiencing less pleasure from the music than those who saw the same food without the McDonald's packaging. The first group also reported that the music seemed to go on for longer.

The researchers concluded that simply being exposed to fast food symbols reduces people's tendency to savour pleasant experiences and derive happiness from them. The suggestion being that the 'fast' aspect of fast food reflects and reinforces a culture of impatience – subconsciously triggering a need for speed which is incompatible with proper enjoyment of life's simple pleasures.

Happiness hint ☑

Avoid looking at anything to do with fast food.

My most recent ex-boyfriend described McDonald's as 'filth', to which I liked to reply, 'Takes one to know one!'

But to be honest, he was right: eating fast food is enjoyable at the time but makes you feel grubby afterwards, much like having casual sex or watching trashy TV like *Love Island* – so it doesn't surprise me one bit that junk food dulls the senses and impedes pleasurable experiences.

The way I see it, humans have two basic modes of behaviour, which I'll call 'easy' and 'hard'. 'Easy' mode is doing stuff you know *isn't* good for you but *feels* good while you do it, including all of the following:

- Eating crappy food full of fat and sugar that's devoid of any nutrients

- Having sex with someone you don't love

- Binge-watching reality TV shows or reading trashy bonkbusters

- Spending all day browsing social media

- Lying on the couch instead of exercising, as per the last chapter

- Doomscrolling on your phone instead of paying attention to your kids

'Hard' mode is the opposite: doing stuff that may feel less immediately enjoyable but which gives you a better future:

- Eating healthy food

- Exercising (I know, I know)

- Having a loving long-term relationship instead of one-night stands with people you don't care about

- Reading literary fiction or a broadsheet

- Switching off electronic devices to spend quality time with your kids playing board games

There's a wise saying: 'The easy way now produces a hard way later; the hard way now produces an easy way later.' If you eat a lot of junk food, I reckon it's difficult to feel good about yourself, as you know you're wrecking your health and weight. At the same time, watching other people eat Krispy Kreme Doughnuts while you're chowing down on broccoli is no fun.

So do as I say, not as I do. And remind yourself that you're gonna live longer and feel happier in the long run.

Reference:

House J., DeVoe S.E., Zhong C.B., Too Impatient to Smell the Roses: Exposure to Fast Food Impedes Happiness. *Soc Psychol Personal Sci.* 2014;5(5):534–41.

The Happiness Interview: Andrew Copson

Andrew Copson is Chief Executive of Humanists UK and President of Humanists International. Together with Alice Roberts, he wrote The Sunday Times *bestseller* The Little Book of Humanism *(Piatkus, 2020).*

What three things make you happiest?

Drinking and eating with friends.

Reading novels.

Cuddling with my dog.

What three things would make you happier?

Perfect health.

An unlimited library.

Enormous wealth with which to buy all my friends everything they ever wanted, fund all the charitable works I could think of, and live my whole life in comfort.

What advice would you give to anyone who wants to be happy?

When I reflect on why I am content I think it is because I have things to do (worthwhile work and interesting hobbies) and people to love (friends, 'god'children, my partner). This not only makes me happy in the here and now but gives me things to look forward to, which I think must be an additional ingredient of happiness. So my advice would be – find those things! And cultivate a positive outlook on things, not worrying too much. We can choose to be happy, within limits, so make the choice!

Chocolate

Research study 📁

Title: The Sweet Life: The Effect of Mindful Chocolate
   Consumption on Mood

Year: 2017

Country: USA

Chocolate has been the subject of plenty of research studies and lots of us find pleasure in eating it, so it was only a matter of time before scientists decided to test out its effect on happiness. A small number of studies had been published previously which linked chocolate consumption with improved mood and reduced anxiety, but this one went a step further by also testing the effect on mood of eating chocolate in a state of mindfulness.

The concept of mindfulness is rooted in Buddhist philosophy. It places an emphasis on focusing on the present environment and having a receptive, non-judgemental awareness of one's feelings and experiences in the moment. Some individuals may strive to achieve a high state of mindfulness in their lives as the norm. One doesn't have to be a generally mindful person, however, in order to adopt a mindful state in a particular moment.

In this experiment, participants were randomly assigned to one of four groups. Two groups ate a small amount of chocolate and the other two groups ate plain crackers. For each food, one group was directed to adopt a mindful state while eating and the other wasn't. The mood of every participant was measured before and after they'd eaten. They weren't told that the study was testing the effect of mindfulness, in case this biased their responses. The participants were 273 college students, 167 of whom were female, with an average age of nineteen. Some received fifteen dollars for taking part, while others received credit on their course.

Before eating either the chocolate or the crackers, all participants listened to one of two short audio recordings. Those in the mindfulness groups heard a recording which instructed them to eat the food slowly, hold it in their hands and gaze at it, think about the farmers who'd produced the ingredients, and focus on the sensations of putting it in their mouths. Before and after eating, they all answered various sets of questions designed to measure mood. At the end of the experiment, they also answered questions for measuring mindfulness and how much they'd liked the food.

The results showed that those who'd eaten the chocolate experienced a boost to their mood which wasn't shared by those who'd eaten the crackers. In addition, the mindful chocolate-eaters benefitted from a greater mood boost than the non-mindful chocolate-eaters. For those who ate the crackers, there was no benefit to mindful eating.

The researchers noted that this fitted with an existing theory that being in a mindful state can enhance positive experiences. They concluded that, for those who find it pleasurable, eating chocolate induces a state of greater happiness, but doing it in a mindful way increases the effect. They also noted that the quantity of chocolate consumed was relatively small (approximately a third of a standard sized chocolate bar), so large quantities don't need to be consumed to make people feel better.

The experiment doesn't tell us whether eating a larger amount of chocolate would cause a larger boost to happiness or how long the uplift in mood lasts after eating. It's also possible that the same results would apply to eating any food which someone finds pleasurable and that there's nothing particularly special about chocolate (apart from the fact that lots of people enjoy eating it).

Happiness hint ☑

Eat small amounts of chocolate (if you like it) for a quick happiness boost and enter a mindful state while doing it if you want to get the maximum effect.

I'm going out with a man who is allergic to chocolate, which has to be the world's worst allergy (except for those people who are allergic to air and water). I am a chocoholic so, selfishly, my first thought was, 'At least he won't try to share mine!'

Maybe the mindfulness thing works because it takes longer for the chocolate to melt in your mouth if you eat it slowly, so you get to experience the taste sensation for longer? You're actively appreciating the stuff rather than bolting it down in a hurry.

Chocolate is a lot nicer than crackers, so I can see why it would make you happier. I read another study showing that cocoa makes you release endorphins, and that the darker the chocolate, the more cocoa it contains and the more endorphins you release. Shame it's so bitter, as that would offset the feel-good chemicals for me.

A third of a standard sized chocolate bar is nowhere near enough, by the way. I like to wolf down those 200g bars of Dairy Milk, which is why I'm currently a big mama whose arse has its own postcode.

Reference:
Meier B.P., Noll S.W., Molokwu O.J., The sweet life: The effect of mindful chocolate consumption on mood. *Appetite*. 2017;108 (September):21–7.

Beauty

Research study 🗀

Title: Beauty is the Promise of Happiness?

Year: 2013

Country: Various

We live in a society that places such a high value on physical attractiveness that we often assume that beautiful people must be happier people. In this study, US researchers set out to discover whether those who are considered better-looking really do feel more happy. They used existing data on beauty and happiness from four countries – Canada, Germany, the UK and the US. As there is no standard way to measure beauty for research purposes (and different ways to measure happiness), they deliberately chose data from surveys in which different methods had been used. They did this to make it more likely that any relationship between beauty and happiness showing in their analysis was reflective of something that occurs in the real world, rather than simply being due to the quirks of one particular measurement technique.

The researchers theorised that beauty could affect happiness through two mechanisms – the direct effect on one's wellbeing of feeling attractive in itself and the indirect effect that may come from experiencing advantages in life afforded to good-looking people. There is evidence, for example, that physical attractiveness increases success in the job market.

159

One set of US data came from the Quality of American Life surveys undertaken in 1971 and 1978. Random samples of the US adult population were asked questions by an interviewer who also assessed each participant's looks on a scale of one to five. More data from the US was taken from the Wisconsin Longitudinal Survey, which followed a group of high-school graduates from 1957. The assessment of the participants' beauty in this case came from showing their high-school graduation photos to a panel of people in 2004 and asking them to rate each one. The panel had an even split of men and women, nearly all of whom were older than the participants – meaning that they had an awareness of what good looks were considered to be in the late 1950s. The participants were interviewed at age fifty-three and again at age sixty-five and asked questions to rate their happiness.

Canadian data was taken from the Quality of Life (QOL) survey, which occurred every two years from 1977 to 1981 with a sample of the adult population. Again, an interviewer asked participants a wide range of questions and rated their looks on a five-point scale. The same participants were rated each time the survey was conducted but the interviewers changed, generating three independent ratings of each person's beauty.

The German data came from the General Social Survey conducted in 2008. In this survey the interviewer rated the participants' looks both at the start and end of the interview using an eleven-point scale.

UK data was taken from the British National Child Development Study, which followed a cohort of children born in 1958. When they were aged seven and eleven, each child had their physical attractiveness rated by his or her teacher. At ages thirty-three, forty-one, forty-six and fifty-one, those who were still participating in the study were asked questions to measure how happy they were.

> When they analysed the data they'd brought together, the researchers found that happiness was increased by physical beauty. They concluded that at least half of this increase was down to indirect benefits of beauty – better-looking people tending to do better in the job market and to marry people with higher incomes. These indirect benefits accounted for a greater proportion of the beauty-happiness boost experienced by men compared to women. The results of the study also showed that females' looks were rated more extremely than males.

Happiness hint ☑

Be beautiful.

I'm currently a hot girl trapped in a fat girl, so I've experienced being both conventionally pretty and conventionally ugly. There are definitely huge differences in the way you're treated by society.

When you're pretty, guys stop their cars to let you cross the street so they can watch you walk by, even if it's not a zebra crossing. When you're ugly, guys drive into you even if it *is* a zebra crossing! It's like they think you're invisible, or at least unworthy of nice treatment.

I also found it far easier to get jobs when I was conventionally pretty – and, of course, boyfriends.

There's a dark flip side to this, though: when I was skinny and beautiful, I was sexually assaulted more times than I could count. Since piling on the weight, it's only happened once, so there are benefits to being invisible.

When I realised that guys only wanted to date me when I was skinny and not when I was fat, I became extremely disillusioned with relationships. Especially when it came to a guy who I'd been friends with for years; I was the only girl ever to sleep with him, and yet he felt within his rights to reject me because, as he put it, 'you weren't taking care of yourself'.

I protested that, surely, if you loved someone and they weren't taking care of themselves, that's the exact time when you should take care of them?

I realised he was an incredibly shallow and superficial person, and that the same was true of a lot of men. When I was slim, I found it easy to get dates on dating apps; when I was fat, it was virtually impossible.

And then I met Kieran, who thinks I'm beautiful whatever I weigh, and doesn't need me to lose or gain weight. He loves me despite my size. He also likes me to look natural, so he doesn't care if I don't wear make-up and he prefers me with natural body hair.

I'd never sent a naked selfie before I met him, because I'd always felt so self-conscious about my brown nipples and dark vagina. My body was so different from those of other women I'd seen naked. But Kieran thinks I'm the hottest girl ever, and that seems to transcend my appearance.

I'm so glad I found him.

Reference:
Hamermesh D.S., Abrevaya J., Beauty is the Promise of Happiness? *Eur Econ Rev.* 2013;64:351–68.

The Happiness Interview: Count Binface

Count Binface is an intergalactic space warrior, part-time politician and officially London's ninth choice to be mayor of the Earth Capital, after the 2021 election in which he defeated the twin evils of Piers Corbyn and UKIP. He has challenged two British Prime Ministers at general elections: Theresa May in 2017 and Boris Johnson in 2019 (the former in his previous guise as Lord Buckethead). Count Binface offers strong, not entirely stable leadership, and he won't rest until Ceefax is restored, London Bridge is renamed 'Phoebe Waller', and no croissant costs more than £1. Sensible policies for a happier Britain.

What three things make you happiest?

Conquering alien planets, people spelling my name correctly (the 'o' is very important), *Lovejoy*, and subverting questions like this with a super-fluous fourth answer.

What three things would make you happier?

One: Conquering Earth (which is a work in progress, I'll grant you).

Two: The return of Ceefax and all other Teletext-based news services, which I will introduce to Britain within the first hundred days of taking power.

Three: Making Piers Morgan zero emissions by 2030, another of my flagship policies.

What advice would you give to anyone who wants to be happy?

I suggest that the quickest route to being 'Happy' is to write a catchy dance-pop ditty with that very title. It might make other people slightly less happy each time they hear it, but the odds are that your financial problems will be over. That's how to achieve material happiness. As for satisfying your soul, that's easy: vote Count Binface!

Part 4: Outlook on life

Sense of humour

Research study 🗀

Title: Humor Styles, Self-Esteem, and Subjective Happiness

Year: 2014

Country: Hong Kong

We tend to associate laughter with happiness, so it might seem natural to assume that people with a good sense of humour would be happier than those without one. Humour comes in different forms, however – some of them positive and some negative. Those with an 'affiliative' style of humour tend to make jokes or spontaneously engage in witty banter in order to create amusement, reduce tension when interacting with others and help build relationships. People with a 'self-enhancing' sense of humour tend to find amusement in everyday incongruities. Types of humour which are classed as 'maladaptive' include aggressive humour and self-defeating humour. Previous research has shown that these are more common among men than women.

Those who use aggressive humour make fun of other people in order to amuse themselves or others, while those who use self-defeating humour make fun of themselves.

This study investigated the relationship between different styles of humour, happiness and self-esteem among undergraduate students in Hong Kong. The researchers recruited 135 women and 92 men from the same university. They were aged from eighteen to twenty-eight, with an average age of twenty-one. The participants completed a questionnaire on humour styles and a standard set of questions designed to measure happiness.

The results showed that affiliative and self-enhancing humour styles were both linked with higher self-esteem and happiness. There was no significant relationship between greater use of maladaptive humour and levels of self-esteem or happiness.

Although the researchers were able to demonstrate that happy students with high self-esteem tended to use more affiliative and self-enhancing humour, rather than making fun of others or themselves, the study doesn't prove that this actually causes people to be happier. We also can't assume that it would show the same results if it were replicated with participants from different age groups and cultures. Its findings do, however, fit with evidence from other studies that these types of humour help with building social support and developing a positive mindset.

Happiness hint ☑

If you tend to primarily make jokes at the expense of yourself or other people, consider switching to a more positive style of humour.

Arrgh, I hate it when blokes rip the piss out of me. Like, I'd rather they do it in front of me than behind my back like girls often do, but still – it's mean and unnecessary.

Thankfully, Kieran has never done this, and John knows better than to do this now because I've menaced him, mwahahaha. But guys do seem to bond through slagging each other off. It's perplexing.

You might expect me, as a comedy writer and former stand-up, to feel sanguine about people telling all kinds of jokes, even jokes at my expense. But there's a huge difference between telling jokes at a comedy club and in real life. People are more willing to accept being made fun of if they've gone out to a club for the night and it's part of the show, whereas they're far less willing to be made fun of in their own front room by someone who isn't a professional comedian.

And there are even limits to comedy shows: if a comic goes too far and rips the piss out of an audience member mercilessly for no reason, the audience can easily turn against that comic – because bullying in the name of humour is still bullying.

Lily is at the stage where she tells jokes like, 'What do you call a sleeping bull? A bulldozer!' Now that's the kind of humour I can get on board with.

Reference:
Yue X.D., Wing-Yin K.L., Jiang F., Hiranandani N.A., Humor Styles, Self-Esteem, and Subjective Happiness. *Psychol Rep.* 2014;115(2):517–25.

Compassion

Research study 🗁

Title: Practicing Compassion Increases Happiness and Self-Esteem

Year: 2010

Country: Canada

The capacity to experience compassion requires empathy, sympathy and a sense of caring for other people. As a key building block of healthy human relationships, we tend to regard compassion as a desirable psychological trait to be encouraged and applauded. Evidence indicates that as well as benefitting others, being a compassionate person may also have benefits for the individual, including higher self-esteem and a reduction in symptoms of depression.

In this study, researchers conducted an experiment to test whether compassionate behaviour led to a change in happiness, self-esteem and levels of depression. They recruited participants through Facebook ads which invited Canadian adults to take part in what was described as an online study exploring the effect of positive exercises on mood. A total of 719 people were signed up for the study. Their ages ranged from seventeen to seventy-two, with an average age of thirty-three. Over 80% were female. The participants were paid thirty dollars if they completed week one. The reward for continuing after this point was entry into various prize draws throughout the duration of the study.

Firstly, they provided basic information about themselves and completed a set of questionnaires designed to measure their levels of happiness, self-esteem, depression and romantic attachment. The participants were randomly divided into two groups. One group was instructed to behave compassionately towards another person every day for a week. They were told to actively help or interact with someone in a supportive and considerate way, and given examples such as 'talking to a homeless person' or 'simply being more loving to those around you'. Each evening they had to go online to log the day's compassionate experience. The second group were given a non-compassionate task to provide a neutral comparison. They were instructed to engage in a daily psychological exercise for a week involving describing an early memory and to spend ten minutes each night writing about that memory in as much detail as possible. After seven days, both groups completed the questionnaires again and on three more occasions over the following six months.

The analysis of the questionnaire data showed that those in the compassion group experienced sustained increases in their levels of happiness and self-esteem over six months that were not experienced by those in the neutral comparison group. This finding fitted with previously published research suggesting that being compassionate is good for one's mental wellbeing.

The researchers speculated that undertaking compassionate actions may have helped to give people a greater sense of meaning and purpose in their lives and that this in turn led to an increase in happiness.

Happiness hint ☑

Be a compassionate person and actively seek out opportunities to show compassion towards others every day.

I use a meditation app called Balance, and one of the meditations I practise with it is called Loving-Kindness. One morning, the app asked me to wish for something good for a stranger, so I wished that the man who managed the checkouts at Poundland would have a good day.

Later that day, I saw him and he looked very grumpy, so the meditation clearly hadn't worked!

But anyhow, it makes sense to me that being compassionate would make you happier. Everyone wants to feel good about themselves, and if you're a nice person who tries to make life better for others, it stands to reason that you'd have higher self-esteem and feel happier than if you acted like a dick.

I guess the explanation about having a greater sense of purpose and meaning in your life checks out too. I'm a lot happier for being a mother, and just want to fill my daughter's life with joy, so that's given me more reason for being here. Of course, I'm not compassionate 24/7, because it's tricky when she yells 'I HATE you!' in my face, but I genuinely try to always remain calm and to think of her feelings. As a result, we're really close and have a strong, very loving bond between us, and there's nothing better in the world.

Who are you most compassionate to, and why?

Reference:
Mongrain M., Chin J.M., Shapira L.B., Practicing Compassion Increases Happiness and Self-Esteem. *J Happiness Stud.* 2011;12(6):963–81.

Gratitude

Research study 🗀

Title: Gratitude Predicts Hope and Happiness:
      A Two-study Assessment of Traits and States

Year: 2018

Country: USA

A trait we often associate with happy people is the ability to recognise, and feel thankful for, the positive things that have happened in their lives. Gratitude is the feeling of appreciation we get when we know that we've benefitted from something given to us by another person. As well as physical objects, this could be less tangible things such as help, advice, kindness or emotional support. It's not restricted to things explicitly given as gifts, but can apply to anything good that we've received from others.

This two-part study explored the relationship between gratitude, happiness and hope for the future.

Firstly, 181 undergraduate college students from a liberal arts college in the US Midwest were recruited to complete a survey in return for course credit. Most were female and their ages ranged from seventeen to twenty-seven, with an average age of twenty. The survey assessed various personality traits and included questions designed to measure hope, gratitude, forgiveness, patience, self-control and happiness over the past month.

Analysis of the data showed that those with a more grateful disposition tended to also be happier. It turned out that gratitude was a better predictor of happiness than forgiveness, patience and self-control combined.

For the second part of their investigation, the researchers recruited 153 students from the same college. Their ages ranged from fifteen to twenty-three, with an average age of nineteen. Again, the majority were female.

They were first asked to write about a specific outcome they were hoping to experience in the future and which was partly out of their control. They were also asked to describe how they would feel if this hope came to fruition and to hold this in their minds while their levels of current hope and happiness were measured. The participants were then randomly split into two groups. One group were asked to describe a past hope that had been fulfilled. In order to provide a neutral comparison, the other group were asked to describe their travelling routes on the previous day. At this point, measures were again taken of the participants' levels of hope for the desired outcome they'd thought of originally and their current happiness.

The results of this experiment showed that gratefully remembering a past hope that had come to fruition increased hope and happiness. Those who were assigned to the neutral comparison group did not experience the same effect.

There are limitations on how much we can conclude from this because participants weren't representative of the make-up of the general population and the experiment only measured the effect in the very short term. We don't know how long this uplift in people's feelings of hope and happiness lasted after the experiment was over. The study provides credible evidence, though, that adopting a grateful mindset may help to increase happiness.

Happiness hint ☑

Have an attitude of gratitude.

Grateful is basically the opposite of bitter. You can't feel angry and miserable at the same time as expressing thanks for all the good things you have, because they're diametrically opposing emotions.

Focus on good things, feel happy. Focus on shit things, feel awful. It's an easy, simple choice and yet so many of us unwittingly choose the latter.

Of course, if something crap has just happened to you, you often need to vent and let it out. Pretending it hasn't happened isn't necessarily healthy. But when people hang on to stuff that happened years ago and continue moaning about it, it's time to sing that song from *Frozen*.

I don't have all the answers. I'm the woman who doesn't forgive, remember? But in my day-to-day life, I'm broadly fairly happy, and I think that's because I know how lucky I am to have Lily, and Kieran, and John, and all the other wonderful people I know.

I'm grateful that I have my own house, and the ability to create for a living. The chance to influence the world with my music, art and words – you're reading them right now! – which is a kind of immortality, unless every single copy of my books gets burnt.

I'm grateful for my health, safety, everything I own, and the opportunity to be alive right now. Hell, better to be alive in 2022 than 1022, with its lack of dentistry and pop music.

And being grateful for all this doesn't mean denying that I had a shit childhood. I can simultaneously acknowledge this and be grateful that it's over, and that unlike many people who had traumatic childhoods, I'm not on the streets, on drugs, in prison or dead.

What are you most grateful for?

Reference:
Witvliet C. van O, Richie F.J., Root Luna L.M., Van Tongeren D.R., Gratitude Predicts Hope and Happiness: A Two-study Assessment of Traits and States. *J Posit Psychol.* 2019;14(3):271–82.

The Happiness Interview: Jon Holmes

Jon Holmes is a multi-award-winning writer, satirist, presenter and producer. His Radio 4 show The Skewer *has notched up shelfloads of international awards, and his spoof true-crime podcast* Cold Case Crime Cuts *was a recent New York Festival winner and Rose d'Or nominee. He's hosted his own shows on BBC 6 Music, Xfm, 5 Live, LBC, Radio X, Virgin and (a long time ago when he was young) Radio 1. He's since covered Saturday mornings and weekday breakfast on Radio 2, and worked on TV with the likes of Armando Iannucci and Harry Hill. He co-created Radio 4's* Dead Ringers, *and has won Baftas for his work on TV's* Horrible Histories. *He is also an award-winning travel writer, which has seen him arrested in Texas, crocodile hunting in Papua New Guinea, and hospitalised by a colony of sea urchins off the coast of Puerto Rico. His largely uncalled-for memoir* A Portrait of an Idiot as a Young Man *is published by Orion.*

What three things make you happiest?

Three French hens. Frankly, I have no truck with two turtledoves, and four calling birds is too many calling birds. The noise is unbearable. So it's French hens. Three of them. Three is, after all, the magic number, and that also applies to French hens. You can also keep your five gold rings, and shove any sort of singular game bird/deciduous shrub combination up your pipe. Hens x three. That's the happy sweet spot.

What three things would make you happier?

You'd think I'd say another three French hens, wouldn't you? But no. That would be six French hens in total and, as we've established, that is unacceptable. Three is obviously perfect. Why else would there be three condoms in a packet? I don't make the rules, but obviously someone somewhere has stipulated that the number of times one should attempt intercourse in one sitting (or standing, or from behind) is three. To be clear, I am not condoning sex with hens. Save that kind of filth for the milking maids or leaping lords – whatever is your bag. Or drumming drummers. NOTE: be sure to check that they are not *chicken* drummers. Do not have sex with chicken drummers because you will get breadcrumbs in your foof and/or penis. Also, do not have sex with three French hens. Or seven swimming swans. Or even – despite what you might have heard – six geese a-laying. It's not *that* kind of laying. What's wrong with you?

What advice would you give to anyone who wants to be happy?

Hen's eggs.

Authenticity

Research study 🗁

Title: Does Authenticity Predict Subjective Happiness?

Year: 2014

Country: Turkey

The concept of 'being yourself' or 'being true to yourself' is commonly talked about as a desirable trait and a goal for self-development. People who are perceived not to be 'authentic' or 'genuine' are often seen in a bad light because of it, often being labelled as 'fake' or 'false' if the perception is sufficiently negative.

It's not always clear what is meant by 'authenticity' in practical terms, as there is no universally accepted definition of the concept. One idea splits it into three dimensions – degree of self-alienation, acceptance or rejection of external influence, and authentic living. Self-alienation is about having an inadequate sense of one's own identity through lack of understanding and a discrepancy between conscious awareness and real experience. Too much acceptance of external influence is underpinned by a belief that one must change to fit other people's expectations. Authentic living is about behaving in a way that is consistent with one's own beliefs and values.

This study explored the question of whether living life authentically is linked with greater happiness, using this three-component conceptualisation of authenticity. The researcher recruited 317 university students who volunteered to take part. There were slightly more women than men in the study, with participants' ages ranging from seventeen to thirty-one and an average age of twenty-one. They each answered two standard sets of questions designed to measure happiness and the three components of authenticity.

Analysis of the data collected showed that those who were happier tended to be more authentic, based on the definition applied – they were less accepting of external influence, had less self-alienation and were living in a way that was more consistent with their own beliefs and values.

The study had a number of limitations. It only looked at university students and collected data on a single occasion, so we can't say whether the same results would be seen in other sections of the population or whether the relationship between authenticity and happiness remains consistent at different points in time. The study also doesn't tell us whether being more authentic makes people happier or vice versa. It could be that authenticity and happiness simply go together and are both caused by other factors. There's also a possibility that cultural differences in how authenticity is valued might produce different results in other countries. Although it left lots of questions unanswered, the study provides some evidence that being inauthentic could be bad news for achieving happiness.

Happiness hint ☑

Live your values and don't fake who you are to meet other people's expectations.

I feel a bit vindicated by this, because I am always 'myself' – meaning that, when among adults, I am rude, sweary, filthy and have a predilection for TMI disclosures.

This, you'll be amazed to hear, does not please everyone. A regressive man on Twitter recently responded to one of my sweary tweets, telling me that proper ladies shouldn't swear.

I replied, 'Oh gosh, I'm so glad you told me! I hadn't realised. What do proper ladies do? Should I not touch my vagina any more? Perhaps I shouldn't let men touch it either unless we're married? I'll throw out skirts that end above the knee and tops below the neck. More advice needed!'

He retorted that, though *I* clearly thought it was funny, real men wouldn't.

I came back, 'Oh, my dude, it *is* funny. *Very* funny. And real men can handle real women, in all our sweary, filthy, badass glory. You must be an absolute riot in bed my friend. Me: "Fuck my tight wet cunt hard and fast, ohhh yes baby!" You (covering ears): "Noooooooooo, you're not a *proper lady*!"'

(My new friend didn't bother responding to this – wisely, I think.)

The thing is, if you're faking your personality, no one's ever going to like you for you, because they don't *know* you. If you're pretending to be different, it can only be because you think the real you is somehow insufficient or unpalatable – and those negative thoughts are going to adversely affect your self-esteem.

I'm not talking about changing your behaviour here. There are instances in life when you realise you should change the way you act, whether that means you stop gossiping or quit getting into fights with strangers in the street.

No, I'm talking about altering your whole personality: pretending to be an introvert when you're an extrovert, or vice versa. Making out you're conservative when you're liberal, prudish when you're sweary, appalled when you're relieved (or the reverse, in all these situations); basically, acting the opposite of the way you would act if you weren't faking it.

Of course, we all have our politer, more respectful personas activated when we meet a stranger for the first time. We're nicer, more accommodating and more accepting.

But that stranger is never going to become a true friend unless you let them get to know the real you. And, as we know from previous studies, having no true friends is a sad state of affairs.

Reference:
Akin U., Does Authenticity Predict Subjective Happiness? *J Educ Instr Stud World*. 2014;4(2):48–54.

Optimism

Research study 📁

Title: Does Perceived Emotional Intelligence and Optimism/
Pessimism Predict Psychological Well-being?

Year: 2010

Country: Spain

Lifelong pessimists are often thought of as unhappy people, while those with an optimistic outlook may be assumed to feel generally upbeat about their lives. Optimists tend to believe that good things will happen in the future, so it seems logical that they ought to feel happier than people who don't. Building on research showing that pessimism is associated with stress, lower happiness and symptoms of depression, this study set out to explore whether optimism and psychological wellbeing are really linked.

Using a questionnaire, researchers collected data from 217 undergraduate students at a Spanish university campus. All the students were female, the oldest was twenty-eight and their average age was twenty-one. The questions included standard measures of mood, psychological wellbeing and optimistic or pessimistic disposition.

Analysis of the data showed that those who had a more optimistic disposition tended to have better psychological wellbeing. Greater pessimism, on the other hand, was linked with poorer psychological wellbeing.

The researchers acknowledged that questions remained about exactly how one affects the other and whether the same results would be seen in people other than young female students. Also, it's conceivable that excessive optimism might induce a reckless approach to life that leads to harmful risk-taking. This study doesn't tell us whether more optimism always equates to more happiness, or whether there's an optimum level.

Happiness hint ☑

Look on the bright side and expect good things to happen (but don't get too carried away and blow your life savings on lottery tickets).

I'm an optimist. Sometimes this bites me on the bum, like when I keep expecting certain family members to be nice to me, despite a lifetime of evidence that they generally aren't, and then I call them up and they still aren't, and I'm like, 'Whaaat? How come these people, who are generally not nice to me, are persisting in not being nice to me?!'

Sometimes hope, borne of optimism, can be foolish. As the saying goes, the definition of insanity is doing the same thing again and again and expecting different results.

But the belief 'my family members will be nice to me someday' is inherently more optimistic than the belief 'my family members will never be nice to me, so I should give up on them'.

I think some of my friends are a bit worried that I'm so optimistic as to be delusional. I'm convinced that my pop songs are exceptional enough to be huge hits and that I will be the next big pop superstar, despite being forty-one years old and a single mum. Though they're too polite to say it, I'm pretty sure my mates think I'm having a mid-life crisis and am destined for a psychological crash if I don't make it.

I think they haven't factored in two things: firstly, that my songs are absolute bops. They're incredibly catchy, melodic and danceable (is that a word? It is now) with intelligent lyrics and gorgeous pop production. If they're not massive hits I won't just eat my hat, I'll eat my whole outfit including my trainers, which I suspect to be rather chewy.

And secondly, I'll be doing what I love, so even if I don't hit the dizzy heights of superstardom (which I reckon is probably very stressful anyway) I'll still be having a great time.

And isn't that what life is about?

Reference:
Augusto-Landa J.M., Pulido-Martos M., Lopez-Zafra E.,
Does Perceived Emotional Intelligence and Optimism/Pessimism
Predict Psychological Well-being? *J Happiness Stud.* 2011;12(3):463–74.

Hedonism

Research study 📁

Title: Individualism as the Moderator of the Relationship between Hedonism and Happiness: A Study in 19 Nations

Year: 2016

Country: Various

Hedonism can be thought of as a philosophy of life in which pleasure is valued as an end in itself. While most of us would probably say that we want pleasure in our lives, hedonists are truly devoted to the pursuit of pleasurable experiences and self-gratification.

Researchers from South Korea and New Zealand had a theory that hedonism would be a greater cause of happiness in countries with more individualistic cultures, rather than those with cultures which placed greater emphasis on the group. This idea was based on a large body of evidence showing that an alignment between a person's own values and those of the society they're living in is beneficial for mental wellbeing.

They analysed existing data from the first wave of the International Wellbeing Study, which began in 2009. Across nineteen countries, 6,899 participants completed the same survey a total of five times over the course of a year. In their analysis, the researchers included the results from standard questions in the survey designed to measure people's perceptions of their own happiness and the degree to which they had a hedonistic approach to life. They also used existing figures on national levels of individualism and the overall economic prosperity of the same countries.

The results of their analysis supported their theory. Hedonism was shown to be more strongly correlated with happiness in countries with more individualistic cultures (such as the USA, Australia and UK) than countries with more collectivist cultures (such as Colombia and China). They concluded that adopting a hedonistic approach to life may be a more effective route to happiness in individualistic cultures.

The researchers acknowledged that this finding shouldn't be regarded as conclusive, due to some limitations of their study. Some regions of the world (including Africa and South America) were under-represented in the data. Also, the survey only measured hedonism by asking about people's attitudes to pleasure and not how often they actually engaged in pleasurable activities.

Interestingly, this isn't the first study to show that national culture can influence happiness. Scientists have also demonstrated that countries with either very permissive or very controlled societies tend to have lower levels of happiness and higher suicide rates than those which have a more moderate approach.***

Happiness hint ☑

If you live in a country that primarily values individualism, try being a hedonist.

*** Harrington J.R., Boski P., Gelfand M.J., Culture and National Well-being: Should Societies Emphasize Freedom or Constraint? *PLoS One.* 2015;10(6). doi:10.1371/journal.pone.0127173

Cats have to be the ultimate hedonists. They lie basking in the sun all day, licking their bumholes, then fall asleep.

I am basically a cat, though I don't lick my bumhole (chance would be a fine thing).

Actually, I was a cat once. We had a make-up lady come into school when I was about twelve. She'd done the make-up for Bond films in the 1980s, and she asked if anyone wanted a makeover. The whole hall full of girls put up their hands, and she chose me and turned me into a cat.

When my dad came to collect me from school, I raced into his car and said excitedly, 'Dad, Dad! I was made up by the woman who made up Roger Moore!'

He raised an eyebrow and replied, 'I knew he didn't exist.'

But back to hedonism: what is life without pleasure? I don't take drugs or drink, but great sex and delicious food are what make life worth living – and I'm pretty sure an orgasm a day keeps the doctor away (out of sheer embarrassment, if you wank in close proximity to them).

I admire and yet don't really understand people who lead totally ascetic lives, like my mother, who lives on rice and mung beans. Just thinking of my next meal would make me deeply unhappy.

I'm sure my mum will live into her hundreds while I'll probably conk out at eighty, but I'd rather be a hedonist than abstain from pleasure.

Reference:
Joshanloo M., Jarden A., Individualism as the moderator of the relationship between hedonism and happiness: A study in 19 nations. *Pers Individ Dif.* 2016;94:149–52.

The Happiness Interview: Sanjeev Kohli

Sanjeev Kohli is the co-writer and co-star of award-winning BBC Radio 4 comedy Fags, Mags and Bags, *has written for sketch shows* Chewin' the Fat *and* Goodness Gracious Me, *has presented extensively on the BBC, and has written and recorded vocals for the musical project The Grand Gestures. He has also appeared in the likes of* Cold Feet, Fresh Meat *and* Look Around You *(where he played Synthesizer Patel), as well as being the star of the video for Elbow's 'Lost Worker Bee'. He is best known, however, for playing shopkeeper Navid in* Still Game *for nine series on the BBC and three sell-out runs at The Glasgow Hydro. He is also a keen Twitter enthusiast – he was recently retweeted by Martina Navratilova, which of course had been his long-term plan since 1978. You can follow him at* @govindajeggy.

What three things make you happiest?

Hearing the laughter of my children. (Not when I'm trying to berate them, though, that's straight-up disrespectful and fucking irritating.)

Completing the *Guardian* cryptic crossword. I think I've managed to complete it maybe five or six times in my life, and for about thirty or forty minutes afterwards, I feel UTTERLY indestructible. Those are the narrow time-windows in which I attempt to bleed radiators, invite nephews to 'punch your uncle really hard in the stomach! Come on! Take a run-up' and, on one nearly tragic occasion, fly.

My mum's lamb curry accompanied by her diaphanous chapattis. I don't employ the epithet 'diaphanous' lightly. They're practically ephemeral. Nearly not actually there. I once inhaled NINE in one sitting.

What three things would make you happier?

A world where inner beauty equated to outer beauty.

Completing the *Guardian* cryptic crossword with Stephen Fry. It would be a damned sight quicker; I would get to hang out with Stephen Fry, and he would be there to use his mellifluous tones to convince me not to try flying again.

GENUINELY SPREADABLE butter. And I mean straight from the fridge.

What advice would you give to anyone who wants to be happy?

Lower your goals. Or, rather, ration your goals. So, for example, instead trying to end world hunger, offer a peckish-looking stranger a French Fancy.

Smiling

Research study 🗁

Title: Smiling Makes Us Happier: Enhancing Positive Mood and
     Communication with Smile-encouraging Digital Appliances

Year: 2011

Country: Japan

Smiling is probably regarded as the most obvious and basic sign of happiness, but some research has suggested that the act of smiling can actually improve our mood rather than just being an indicator that someone is already feeling happy. This has been found to be the case even when the smiling is forced or disingenuous. Inspired by this, scientists in Japan created and tested out a machine designed to encourage people to smile more often. Their device, called HappinessCounter, was intended to help people to realise when they're low in mood throughout the day and nudge them into smiling in order to lift their spirits. They felt this would be particularly helpful for people living alone who don't have the benefit of someone around to point out to them when they're not smiling.

The device consists of a digital camera, an LED matrix display and a light sensor, and can be mounted behind a one-way mirror or attached to another surface which the user will be facing regularly in the course of their day. If the device detects a smile it keeps a record and provides visual feedback to the user by displaying an icon of a smiley face.

If insufficient smiling is detected by the device it displays an icon of a sad face. The system could be used in two modes – 'Smile Awareness' and 'Smile Gateway'. The first mode is simply set up to alert people to whether they're smiling or not, while the second goes one step further and provides disincentives for not smiling, e.g. by making it harder to open a door or turn on the TV until a smile is detected.

To test out the impact of the system, the scientists set it up in two homes – one occupied by a person living alone and the other by a couple living together. In both houses, the HappinessCounter device was attached to the refrigerator for ten days. When insufficient smiles were detected, the device was able to make the fridge door more difficult to open by way of a magnet. The participants were asked to use the fridge as they would do normally for the duration of the experiment and to record their feedback on the system by keeping a daily diary.

The scientists concluded that the system had been a success, with both households reporting that it had caused them to smile more and improved their mood. It was noted that at first, the participants' smiles when approaching the fridge seemed somewhat forced but appeared more natural in time as they got used to it. All expressed privacy concerns about the device's camera, given that they commonly went to the fridge after getting out of the bath.

The practicality of installing such a system for everyday use on a large scale is questionable and, as only three participants were used in the experiment, the results don't tell us how effective it would be for different types of people. We also don't know whether the system would continue to be effective for longer periods, or if people would simply come to ignore the device in time outside the context of a research study. The experiment does, however, provide some further evidence to suggest that forcing ourselves to smile more, even when there's nothing to smile about, could help to improve the way we feel.

> **Happiness hint** ☑
>
> Don't wait until you're happy to smile – smile if you want to get happy (even if you have to fake it).

I think I'd feel a bit odd walking round the house by myself, smiling at nothing and nobody. When I'm out and about and pass a stranger, I do tend to smile at them, though only if it's just us and the street's not crowded. It would be a bit weird to smile at a random stranger in a crowd!

What I didn't understand about the study was that the participants all expressed privacy concerns about the device's camera as they 'commonly went to the fridge after getting out of the bath'.

Let's repeat that: they went straight to the fridge naked after having a bath.

Why would you do that? Step dripping out of the bath and head straight for the fridge, only to have to fake-smile at it because otherwise it won't open?! Personally, I put my clothes on after having a bath, but maybe that's just me.

Maybe they'd had a super-hot bath and fancied a cold drink afterwards, but I found it baffling and hilarious.

You might even say it made me smile.

Reference:

Tsujita H., Rekimoto J., Smiling makes us happier: Enhancing positive mood and communication with smile-encouraging digital appliances. *UbiComp'11 – Proc 2011 ACM Conf Ubiquitous Comput.* 2011:1–10. doi:10.1145/2030112.2030114

Mindfulness

Research study 🗀

Title: Meditation and Happiness: Mindfulness and Self-compassion
   May Mediate the Meditation–Happiness Relationship

Year: 2016

Country: Spain

The practice of mindfulness has become a common way that people try
to improve their mental wellbeing. Mindfulness is all about paying
attention to your experiences in the present moment – noticing the
things around you and your own thoughts and feelings on a deeper
level. Mindful people have a heightened awareness of simple pleasures
and sensations that we might normally take for granted or ignore as we
live our busy lives – such as the taste of our food or the feeling of
objects against our skin. There are various types of classes, interventions
and meditation courses aimed at people who want to develop a more
mindful way of being.

Having a mindful disposition has been shown to be associated with
lower levels of stress and anxiety, as well as positive emotions and
greater satisfaction with life. Mindfulness has also been found to be
linked with self-compassion. Having self-compassion is about being in
touch with your own suffering, rather than blocking it out or discon-
necting from it, and having the conscious desire to heal that suffering

by being kind to yourself, rather than blaming or punishing yourself. It's been suggested that mindfulness and self-compassion can go together – enabling and strengthening each other. Self-compassion has also been linked with better mental health, including lower anxiety and stress. This study sought to explore the relationship between happiness, meditation, mindfulness and self-compassion.

Researchers posted a link to an online survey on several Spanish websites about mindfulness, meditation and psychology, as well as social networks, such as Facebook. A total of 365 people completed the survey, of whom 183 were meditators. The survey collected basic information, such as age and sex, and how often the respondents meditated. It also included standard questions designed to measure various facets of mindfulness and self-compassion.

Analysis of the data showed that the more people meditated, the more mindful they were, the more self-compassion they had and the happier they were. The researchers found that one specific aspect of mindfulness (the capacity to pay attention to experiences, such as sensations, thoughts and emotions) and two aspects of self-compassion (self-kindness and feelings of common humanity) partly accounted for the link between meditation and happiness. Although the study doesn't prove that adopting these traits causes people to be happier, the findings add to other evidence which suggests that mindfulness may be beneficial for mental wellbeing. Around two-thirds of the respondents were women, and most were university educated, so we can't be sure if these same results would be seen in a more representative sample of the general population, however.

Happiness hint ☑

Try taking up mindfulness meditation.

Well, I'm a university-educated woman (I hated every second of it, but I did it) so maybe it could work for me?

I know I should meditate more often, but I always forget, because there are so many things in life that are more urgent and pressing: like caring for my daughter, making a living, dieting, etc. Meditation always seems to fall by the wayside.

But, as I mentioned before, I do have an app called Balance which I use when I remember. A man called Ofosu with a wonderfully deep, mellifluous voice talks me through various practices – each session is different.

One practice is called 'body scanning', where you bring your awareness to different parts of your body, relaxing each part in turn. (Ofosu never asks me to bring awareness to my fanny, though, which I think is a notable omission.)

Another practice is 'breath focus', where you concentrate on your breath going in and out of your lungs and chest. It doesn't sound wildly exciting, but it's very relaxing.

I think I do feel better and happier when I meditate. I just need to remember to do it. Maybe Ofosu could implant the suggestion in my brain with his hypnotic voice?

Reference:
Campos D., Cebolla A., Quero S., et al., Meditation and happiness: Mindfulness and self-compassion may mediate the meditation–happiness relationship. *Pers Individ Dif.* 2016;93:80–85.

The Happiness Interview: Bec Hill

Bec Hill has most likely popped up on your TV or Facebook timeline with one of her viral 'paper puppetry' flipcharts (usually demonstrating misheard lyrics). She can also be seen hosting Makeaway Takeaway *on CITV, heard on her podcast* A Problem Squared, *or her words can be read in a series of spooky books called* Horror Heights, *published by Hodder (which are probably available from wherever you got this book from).*

What three things make you happiest?

Hearing children laugh (unless they're ghosts).

Bumping into friends when I least expect it (unless they're ghosts).

Watching movies with a twist at the end (unless I'M a ghost?!).

What three things would make you happier?

More time.

More money.

Fewer ghosts.

What advice would you give to anyone who wants to be happy?

Don't take yourself too seriously. Also, don't become the winter caretaker of an old, isolated hotel.

Trying to be happy

Research study 📁

Title: Trying to be Happier Really Can Work: Two Experimental
    Studies

Year: 2012

Country: USA

One of the most fundamental questions in the field of happiness research is whether trying to be happier is beneficial at all, just as a general principle, regardless of the specific techniques and lifestyle changes which are applied. Some researchers have suggested that trying to be happy could actually be counterproductive. The purpose of this study was to explore this question further, using two different experiments to test out the impact of making a conscious effort to try to be happier on the effect of a happiness-inducing activity.

The activity the researchers chose was listening to music. In the first experiment, they tested differences in how positive people felt depending on both the type of music they listened to and whether they were consciously trying to feel happier at the time. The researchers recruited 173 students from a Midwestern university who were offered course credit in exchange for participating. Some were assigned to listen to part of Stravinsky's *The Rite of Spring*, considered to be mood-neutral, while the others were assigned to listen to part of Copland's *Rodeo*, considered a positively pleasurable piece of music.

Just under half were told to consciously try to improve their mood while listening to the music and the rest were told to avoid any conscious effort to feel happier and simply to listen passively instead. After listening to the music for around twelve minutes they were asked various questions to measure their current mood and ascertain how much they had enjoyed the activity. Data from six of the students had to be discounted because a malfunctioning air conditioner caused the room they were in during the experiment to overheat.

The analysis of this data showed that those who had consciously tried to feel happier and had also listened to the happy music were the happiest of all afterwards. Overall, those who had tried to feel happier and those who hadn't tried to be happier reported enjoying the activity itself to a similar degree. This suggested that the combination of trying to feel happier with an effective practical method for improving happiness produces the optimum result and that the effort of trying to feel happier is not a problematic distraction.

In the second experiment, sixty-eight participants were recruited from a Midwestern liberal arts college and given either cash or extra course credit for participating. They attended five sessions over two weeks in which they listened to music they'd chosen from a selection of genres. Each session lasted fifteen minutes and they had the option of selecting a different genre on each visit. As in the previous experiment, the participants were divided into two groups – with around half told to make a conscious effort to try to become happier over the two weeks and the remainder instructed not to. The groups didn't differ in their level of happiness at the beginning of the experiment. It was made clear that those who were trying to become happier shouldn't engage in any additional activities for the purpose of improving their mood, but simply think about their happiness and try to become happier through their own mental efforts.

After each session, their level of happiness was measured. They also answered questions to measure their appreciation of the selection and quality of music they'd heard, to ensure that this didn't account for any difference in happiness scores between the two groups. Broadly, both groups were equally satisfied with the music offered. The analysis of the data showed that those who'd intentionally tried to become happier experienced an increase in happiness over the two-week period, while the other group did not.

Together, these experiments provide evidence that the conscious pursuit of happiness can be productive, as long as it's accompanied by appropriate practical methods. In other words, just trying to feel happier alone is not enough – you also need to do things that are beneficial for happiness in order to get the full effect. The results also provide evidence that listening to happy music can make you feel happier. A limitation of this study, however, is that it didn't look at the impact of trying to improve your happiness alongside other alternative mood-enhancing activities.

Finally, the researchers considered the question of whether a conscious effort to feel happier is or isn't inconsistent with the practice of mindfulness, in which the focus is on keeping your mind in the present. They concluded that it could be argued either way and that more research was needed.

Happiness hint ☑

Make a conscious effort to try to feel happier in your own mind, as well as doing practical things that make you feel happier. (Also, stop listening to miserable music and swap it for something upbeat.)

Damn that malfunctioning air conditioner! I bet the overheating didn't make those participants feel happier.

But this study is intriguing. I too would have thought actively trying to increase your happiness would be counterproductive, but it turns out we're all wrong. Maybe thinking about happy things you're going to do in the future, things in your life that bring a smile to your face, and happy memories all contribute to making you feel cheerier?

Right now I'm thinking of collecting my daughter from school today, which is bringing me a lot of joy. Even though Lily has asked me to collect her at the corner, because 'If my friends see you, it's embarrassing!'

I pointed out that I'm not *that* uncool a mum, because I'm going to be a huge pop star soon. She retorted, 'Yeah, well, you're not a huge pop star yet, so you're still uncool now!'

But it makes me happy to think of seeing her sweet face, as I don't see her much in the week. I'll take her to a local café and buy her a chocolate brownie and a bottle of juice, and I'll have a cup of tea. We'll play cards and she'll win. She'll tell me all about what she did at school today, and I'll listen, and think, 'How lucky I am to have such a wonderful daughter.'

She makes me the happiest I've ever been.

Reference:
Ferguson Y.L., Sheldon K.M., Trying to be happier really can work: Two experimental studies. *J Posit Psychol.* 2013;8(1):23–3.

Dreaming of a happier future

Research study 🗁

Title: Dreaming of a Brighter Future: Anticipating Happiness
Instills Meaning in Life

Year: 2018

Country: UK

It's natural to assume that hoping for greater future happiness is a key step towards achieving it. Research has shown, however, that people tend to be bad at predicting what will happen to them – painting overly positive pictures of the future in their minds and underestimating the likelihood of bad things occurring. This raises the question of whether dreaming of a happier future is really beneficial or simply means setting ourselves up for disappointment. This final, three-part, study looked at the effect of predicting a brighter future on people's sense that their lives had meaning.

Firstly, the researchers looked at whether imagining an increase in future happiness made people feel that various behaviours in the present were more meaningful. They recruited fifty students on the university campus who volunteered to take part and collected basic information about them. The students' average age was nineteen and most were women. They were divided in two groups, with one group instructed to write down three happy things they anticipated happening in the future and the other instructed to write down any three things they anticipated happening in the future.

Prior to the experiment, the researchers had drawn up a list of twelve behaviours and asked fifteen other students to rank them in order of how instrumental they were in creating happiness. They ranked 'visiting family', 'making friends', 'having a laugh' and 'partying' as most instrumental and 'saving money', 'watching a movie', 'snacking' and 'watching soaps on television' as least instrumental. 'Exercising', 'attending a concert', 'eating healthy' and 'studying' were ranked in the middle.

After they had completed the first exercise, the fifty students were then told to consider the same list of twelve behaviours and rank them in order of how meaningful they were. The results showed that those who'd focused on happy things occurring in the future ranked the behaviours which had been classed as more instrumental to creating happiness as more meaningful compared to those who hadn't. In other words, dreaming of a happy future led to attaching a greater sense of meaning to doing things which were perceived to create happiness.

Secondly, the researchers tested whether people who were more inclined to search for meaning in life also anticipated greater future happiness. They recruited eighty-seven students, most of whom were women, with an average age of twenty-four. The participants completed questionnaires designed to measure their feelings about meaning in life, their current happiness and how happy they expected to be in one to five years' time. Analysis of the data collected showed that those who were searching for meaning in life were particularly inclined to imagine a happier future.

In the final part of the study, the researchers tested whether those who sought meaning in their lives more than others experienced a greater gain in meaning when a state of anticipated happiness was induced.

This time they recruited eighty-two students with an average age of twenty-two – again, the majority were women. The participants completed the 'meaning in life' questionnaire and then, using the same method as in the first experiment, they were split into two groups – one focusing on a happy future and the other on the future in general. They were then asked to what extent they expected their happiness to increase in the future and to what extent they expected their sense of meaning in life to increase in the future. The results demonstrated that those who anticipated a happier future also envisioned a more meaningful life as a consequence. This effect was especially strong among those who were already particularly inclined to seek out meaning in their lives.

Overall, these findings indicate that while imagining a happier future life may cause people to develop unrealistic expectations, it brings the benefit of making their lives seem more meaningful. This raises the question of whether in our quest for happiness the risk of future disappointment is outweighed by the bonus of feeling that life is more meaningful, or vice versa. We know that there's a substantial correlation between happiness and having a sense of meaning in life, but the two things are different and don't always go together. Some happy people have no sense of meaning in their lives, living a selfish and carefree lifestyle. Others may feel that life is very meaningful but are also fairly unhappy, with lives characterised by worry and excessive contemplation.

The relationship between meaning in life and happiness is, therefore, a complex one. It's possible that dreaming of future happiness is overall a good strategy for some people and a counterproductive one for others, depending on the extent to which having meaning in life plays a role in their personal sense of happiness.

Happiness hint ☑

Dreaming of a happier future may set you up for disappointment but may also give your life more meaning. If having meaning in life is important to you, it could be a gamble worth taking.

Daydreaming of a bright future makes me feel happy, regardless of what actually turns out to happen in my life. Because the future is endless, isn't it? As long as you're alive, there's hope of it turning out the way you want.

Granted, you've got to be a little realistic: at the age of forty-one, I'm unlikely to achieve the goal of having more kids, especially as Kieran doesn't want them. But I can alter my goal to that of spending more quality time with the amazing child I already have. That bond between us probably wouldn't be as close or strong with another small child constantly demanding my attention.

When it comes to being a pop star, though, I'm already way past the age most record companies want new artists to be, so it doesn't matter whether I'm forty-two, forty-eight or fifty-five: I'm just as likely or unlikely to make it. And why shouldn't I break the mould and pave the way for great artists who achieve success later in life? The record industry is all about diversity, so why shouldn't this apply to age, too?

My favourite author Helen Dunmore was the same age as me when she published her first novel. Arianna Huffington was fifty-five when she started the *Huffington Post*, fashion designer Vera Wang didn't design a dress until she was forty, and Samuel L. Jackson found fame aged forty-three.

So who's to say you and I won't do the same? You can achieve success at any age, and find love at any age. And even if fertility isn't on your side, you can adopt, foster or mentor children.

Because it would be a sad, small life if we didn't have dreams and goals. I think dreaming of a happier future helps us realise what we need to work towards, and encourages us to be bold and brave and make that imagined future a reality.

So I'll keep dreaming of buying that beautiful glass house in the sunny Hollywood Hills with my royalties from pop stardom, and living in it with Kieran (who will be my husband by then) and daughter Lily (who will have achieved her own dream of becoming a Hollywood actress, fashion designer, author and pop star). I can't think of anything more lovely.

Reference:
van Tilburg W.A.P., Igou E.R., Dreaming of a Brighter Future: Anticipating Happiness Instills Meaning in Life. *J Happiness Stud*. 2019;20(2):541–59.

The Happiness Interview: Arthur Smith

Arthur Smith is a comedian, writer and broadcaster who has appeared on QI, Have I Got News for You *and is best known as the opening bat on* Grumpy Old Men. *He appears regularly on* Loose Ends *on BBC Radio 4, presents* The Comedy Club *on Radio 4 Extra and is the self-proclaimed mayor of Balham and a regular at the Edinburgh Festival since medieval times. His book* 100 Things I Meant to Tell You *(AA Publishing) is out now.*

What three things make you happiest?

I am always chuffed to read a one-star review of a show by someone who is more successful than I am. And I love to read on Twitter that some evangelical Christian antivaxxer I had never heard of has died of Covid. I am also ashamed of the pleasure I take in this kind of *schadenfreude*, which in turn undermines the happiness it affords me. So, instead, here are the three things that make me happiest:

Sleeeeeeep: Every night (and some afternoons), a long soft adventure in which you do no harm, spend no money and have wonderful adventures.

Laughing: 'Laughter is the one true metaphysical consolation' is something Nietzsche might have said. I am always happy laughing with my partner and friends and, as any comedian will tell you, making a roomful of people laugh is a glorious feeling.

Walking: Striding (or these days strolling) along country paths, through woods and trees – or, if need be, along city pavements – is a gift to body and spirit.

What three things would make you happier?

If I could become a koala bear. Koalas sleep for sixteen hours a day and spend their waking hours mooching about and eating with friends. What a life.

If I believed in some beneficent God who answers every question for me.

If Ariane makes millions from this book and gives me some.

What advice would you give to anyone who wants to be happy?

Don't aim too high. Start every day gently by congratulating yourself that you have managed to get up, clean your teeth and put your clothes on not only in the correct order but also the right way round. Well done!

Cultivate acceptance. You can't change the past and, despite what all the inspirational quotes may suggest, you cannot achieve everything you may wish for. Life is a bitch but there are some great bits.

Don't take advice from elderly comedians.

PS Some extra bits:

Think of a good friend you haven't seen for a while, and then send them a postcard. Yes, a proper postcard – with a nice picture on one side and a fond message, an address and a stamp on the other. As you post it imagine your pal receiving it, their pleased face, that smile you have seen so often. Pop into a shop and buy yourself a little edible (or drinkable) luxury, e.g. a slab of your favourite chocolate. Put this to one side . . .

Have a clear-out. Come on, gather up those shoes you know you will never actually wear, the old DVDs, tapes and videos, the chipped teapot, etc., and squash them into that suitcase with the broken wheels. Deposit the whole damn lot in your local charity shop. (NB if your despair is really extreme you could, additionally, throw out a member of your family.) You and your house will feel lighter. And, hey, while you're in the shop, take a quick shufti at the clothes racks – it may be your lucky day . . .

Remember that song you used to love but haven't heard for a while? Yes, that one. Go and stick it on really loud – even if it is 'Lady in Red'. Shut your eyes and, if necessary, dance! As Katie Price once remarked, 'Music hath charms to soothe the glum lady.'

Make a cup of tea. We British know this better than anyone; if in doubt, make a cup of tea.

Turn on the TV, sip your tea, and, for five minutes, watch any reality TV show; savour the beautiful fact that you are not one of the poor saps taking part in it. Then switch the TV off. You have now successfully completed the six activities. It remains only for you to sit quietly and tuck into that little treat you bought after you went to the post box earlier. Oh yes and – why not? – make another cup of tea and, go on with you, take the afternoon off.

Conclusion

We appreciate that there's a shit ton of advice in this book, and thought it might be helpful to recap the main findings. So, to live your best life:

- Be kind to others and yourself. Good, solid, authentic friendships are essential and well worth investing time and effort in. Being big on Twitter or popular on Facebook is no substitute for meaningful connections in the real world.

- Seek out a positive romantic relationship with someone who is similar to you, does their share of the chores around the house and with whom you enjoy great sex. If you find the right person, marry them, but don't marry someone who doesn't fit the bill hoping it will work out, and don't count on having children to elevate your mood.

- Getting to a place where you're financially better off than those around you is likely to make you feel happier, but how much money you have isn't all that matters – how you spend it matters as well. Holidays and fun experiences will give you more happiness in the long run than Versace bags and other material status symbols. If you're not fortunate enough to be financially well off, you can still boost your happiness by investing your time in rewarding relationships and leisure activities.

- It helps to be beautiful, although, of course, we don't all have that luxury. While you can't control your genes, you can still improve the way you feel by adopting a healthy lifestyle.

Conclusion

- To some extent, happiness may be a self-fulfilling prophecy. Smiling, looking on the bright side of life, adopting a positive sense of humour, being grateful for what you have and just making an effort to feel happier have all been shown to have a positive effect on your state of mind.

Go well, and be happy.

Acknowledgements

The authors would like to thank:

All at Little, Brown, especially Andrew McAleer, our fantastic editor, for his steadfast enthusiasm, support, calmness and professionalism.

Stephanie Thwaites and Isobel Gahan at Curtis Brown for their support.

All the celebrities for so generously giving their time and insights for free.

Ariane would also like to thank:

David Conrad for putting in so much hard work and being great fun to work with.

Kieran Byrne for being the kindest, sweetest, most patient and calm friend ever. I'm sorry it didn't work out, but I hope we'll always stay in touch.

John Fleming, aka John Bon Jovial, for being an excellent grandad and great-grandad, and constantly lugging my massive suitcase along on book tours and collecting me from various railway stations around London.

Lucy Spencer for her generosity.

James Harris and Kia Abdullah for our fun chats over coffees.

Lavrentia Foustana for your friendship and amazing proofreading skills. You're a typo-catcher extraordinaire!

Acknowledgements

Andy Davies and all at Taylist Media for giving me the best job ever (Editor of thesethreerooms.com) after I finished this book. Turns out self-employment's not as appealing when you can edit a gorgeous interiors website for a living!

All my incredible Patreon supporters, who generously helped fund the writing process for this book: Peter Weilgony, P.A., Charlie Brooker, Phil Alcock, John Fleming, Lucy Spencer, Dave Cross, Mary and Tim Fowler, Klaas Jan Runia, Mark White, Stef Mo, Kevin McGeary, Dominic McGladdery, Rebekah Bennetch, Keith Bell, Oliver Vass, Steve Richards, Mark Bailey, Matthew Sylvester, Alan Brookland, Marcus P. Knight, Shane Jarvis, Richard Daily, Trevor Prinn, Richard Saunders, Dave Nattriss and Musical Comedy Guide.

And, most of all, my beautiful, hilarious and wonderful Lily – who makes me the luckiest mummy in the whole wide world and universe. I love you to infinity.

Index

elderly people, happiness and
18–19
empathy 170
endorphins 110, 149, 158
ENM (ethically non-
monogamous) 56
exercise 46, 95, 147, 149, 152
extraversion 17

Facebook 37–8
families 94, 138
 see also children; marriage
fast food 150–3
Fincher, David 46
food
 fast food 150–3
 mindful chocolate eating
 156–8
 sharing 13, 19–20, 154
 stockpiling 86
forgiveness 32–4
Forte, Jemma 106–7
friendships
 celebrating friends' successes 31
 having friends you matter to 7–9
 jealousy 5, 30
 old friendships 25
 online friends 11, 12
 real-life friends 10–12
 schadenfreude 30

spending time with friends
15–17
Fry, Stephen 190

goals 14, 25
 dreaming of a happier future
 202–6
 happiness as a moving target 47
 materialistic goals 120, 121
 realistic 190, 208
good news, sharing 29–31
grandchildren 74–6
gratitude 107, 173–6, 211
 predictor of happiness 173–5
grudges 33
Guardian crossword 189, 190

happiness hints
 adopt a healthy lifestyle 109,
 145, 210
 avoid exposure to fast food 151
 avoid pressure to have more sex
 44
 babysit grandchildren 75
 be an optimist 184, 211
 be beautiful 161, 210
 be compassionate 171
 be a (male) swinger 49
 be physically active 148
 boost your income 86

Index

Index